Psychoanalysis and the Struggle for Love

In *Psychoanalysis and the Struggle for Love*, psychiatrist and psychoanalyst Mark Kinet brings together decades of clinical experience, theoretical insight, and cultural curiosity to explore love in all its forms: tender and erotic, destructive and restorative, ancient and digital.

Moving effortlessly between the works of Freud, Lacan, Klein, Winnicott, Balint, Bion, and contemporary neuropsychoanalysis, Kinet reveals how love shapes the psyche from infancy to adulthood, from the consulting room to the wider culture. Across a series of vivid chapters, ranging from early trauma to desire, perversion, seduction, idealisation, digital intimacy, and the healing potential of the analytic setting, this book offers a panoramic portrait of the human need for connection. Kinet combines rigorous clinical thinking with literary and philosophical depth, while offering a clear and compassionate account of why love matters and why it so often goes awry. A compelling exploration of the human heart and the forces that bind us to one another, this is psychoanalysis written with depth, clarity, and warmth.

Written in Kinet's signature engaging and accessible style, this is a vital book for clinicians, readers of mind and culture, and anyone fascinated by the fragile and untidy beauty of love.

Mark Kinet is a psychiatrist, psychotherapist, and psychoanalyst based in Belgium. He is the author of *The Spirit of the Drive in Neuropsychoanalysis* (2023), *Psychoanalytic Principles in Psychiatric Practice: A Remedy by Truth* (2024), *Psychoanalytic Psychotherapy in Psychiatric Practice: Premises and Clinical Portraits* (2025), *Patient Testimonies of Psychodynamic Psychotherapy: Reported and Recorded* (2025), and *The Psychodynamics and Psychogenesis of Parentification* (2026).

'If you want to understand love, Lacan, sex or psychoanalysis, read Kinet!'

Arnon Grunberg, *novelist, essayist, and columnist, Netherlands*

'For Freud, love boiled down to sex, assuming all pleasures arise from a broadly "sexual" drive. For biologists, sex is important because of reproduction; yet, why do we so frequently obtain sexual pleasures in non-procreative ways? In this book – a moving meditation upon love in all its guises – Mark Kinet re-prioritises the mental side, with profound implications for our understanding of the mind's place in Nature: feelings clearly have intrinsic causal powers.'

Mark Solms, *psychoanalyst and neuropsychologist, Professor of Neuropsychology at the University of Cape Town (SA) and founding father of Neuropsychoanalysis*

'These psychoanalytic essays on love's struggles range from Freud to Solms, from Plato to Žižek, traversing deep chasms and celestial heights, from prehistory to science fiction, and from the womb to AI. Their chemistry might disenchant, but their alchemy deepens mystery. A kaleidoscopic perspective opens the reader's mind, also thanks to a style that lucidly names what emerges from darkness. Must read for professionals and lovers.'

Paul Verhaeghe, *emeritus Professor of Psychoanalysis at Ghent University and an internationally acclaimed author*

'*Psychoanalysis and the Struggle for Love* is a sweeping and deeply humane exploration of what it means to love, to desire, and to be recognised. Dr Kinet brings together psychoanalysis, philosophy, and clinical wisdom to illuminate love's generative possibilities and its contradictions. This is a beautifully written, intellectually vibrant book that clinicians and thoughtful readers alike will return to again and again.'

Mark L. Ruffalo, *M.S.W., D.Psa., Assistant Professor of Psychiatry, University of Central Florida College of Medicine, Florida, USA*

'Do *not* read this book by Mark Kinet – because it is too beautiful, too compelling, too accurate. Every chapter, every paragraph, every line, every sentence, like a ballerina, makes a leap and lands on its feet where it makes its point – its *pointe.* Kinet's sentences sharpen our thoughts, honing them until they cut precisely at the place where we believe the matters of love "settle."'

Marc De Kesel, *philosopher and essayist, emeritus Professor at Radboud University Nijmegen (NL) and former associate professor of philosophy at Saint Paul University, Ottawa, Canada*

'*Psychoanalysis and the Struggle for Love* is a wide-ranging meditation on love as the central, conflicted force of our lives. Mark Kinet holds together psychoanalytic insight with philosophy, literature, and clinical sensibility in a voice that is lucid and humane. The result is a book that invites readers to think, and rethink, what loving truly means.'

Arthur Eaton, *PhD, psychoanalyst, journalist, and author based in Amsterdam, Netherlands*

'In *Psychoanalysis and the Struggle for Love*, Mark Kinet brings together philosophy, psychoanalysis, and literature and, in a brilliant, thought-provoking way, shows how love can passionately push people beyond themselves or drag them into catastrophic depths. This is a marvellous book about the many paradoxes of love and, therefore, about what it means to be human.'

Herman Westerink, *Associate and Endowed Professor at the Centre for Contemporary European Philosophy, Radboud University Nijmegen, Netherlands*

Psychoanalysis and the Struggle for Love

A Kaleidoscopic View

Mark Kinet

Routledge
Taylor & Francis Group
LONDON AND NEW YORK

Designed cover image: © The Bubble (2025) by Mieke Teirlinck
https://www.mieketeirlinck.be 50 x 60 cm, Oil on Canvas

First published 2027
by Routledge
4 Park Square, Milton Park, Abingdon, Oxon OX14 4RN

and by Routledge
605 Third Avenue, New York, NY 10158

Routledge is an imprint of the Taylor & Francis Group, an informa business

British Library Cataloguing-in-Publication Data
A catalogue record for this book is available from the British Library

ISBN: 978-1-041-21734-3 (hbk)
ISBN: 978-1-041-21732-9 (pbk)
ISBN: 978-1-003-72876-4 (ebk)

DOI: 10.4324/9781003728764

Typeset in Times New Roman
by KnowledgeWorks Global Ltd.

Contents

1

The Bubble

In trembling hands, a world is spun
not yet self, not yet begun,
a breath of being, barely there,
a sphere of thought, suspended air.

It hums with a caress,
the tender law of more and less:
to hold is loss, to let is keep,
to wake is to disturb the sleep.

The bubble's dreamt in mother's mind,
the reverie that seeks to find
a shape for what cannot be known,
a word, a thought half-grown.

It gleams, an absent core,
the lack that love keeps asking for,
the mirror's ghost, the gaze's plea,
a shimmer of identity.

The silence drifts within,
a pulse beneath the fragile skin
to think is to contain, to bear,
to breathe what breaks, to care...

Again through 'air'.
And when it bursts, the hands remain.
Their emptiness?
The human stain.

Mark Kinet

DOI: 10.4324/9781003728764-1

Prologue

Psychoanalysis and the Struggle for Love

The Struggle for Life

The struggle for life, a well-known phrase that originates in Charles Darwin's theory of evolution, symbolises the constant competition among organisms to survive and reproduce. It is closely linked to the concept of natural selection as the primary driving force of evolution. Just as many Freudian concepts have since entered our everyday language, the term has also become part of it. Where it has permeated the intimate domains of human existence, it is not merely the fight to endure, but the attempt to find form, voice, and coherence amid a world riddled with fragmentation and finitude. In *On the Origin of Species*,[1] Darwin observed that life tends to multiply beyond its means of sustenance, giving rise to a war of all against all, not unlike Thomas Hobbes' infamous brutish realm.[2] But man, unlike the fox or the fern, *suffers* his survival. Man is the only creature who refuses to be what he is, Albert Camus mused.[3] To struggle is not only to stay alive, but foremost to make *sense* of that very act of staying alive.

Sigmund Freud took the battle inward, identifying in the human psyche a conflict between Eros (the warm principle of cohesion and love) and Thanatos (the cold pull towards quietude and return to the inanimate state).[4] In his structural model, the mind is always in conflict, and the Ego has to navigate between the chaos of drives in the Id, the do's and don'ts of the Superego and the armies of reality.[5] This drama is played not on a battlefield, but in dreams, slips, and silences. To be human is to oscillate between creation and collapse.

In developmental psychology, attachment theory offers insight into the early relational roots of psychological well-being and survival. John Bowlby posited that a secure attachment with a caregiver is critical for the child's emotional regulation and resilience.[6] When children are exposed to neglect, abuse, or emotional parentification, they often adapt through survival strategies that may compromise long-term well-being.[7] These early adaptations are part of the struggle to maintain psychological coherence amid emotional threat.

The Meaning of Life

Jacques Lacan, the oracular theorist of language and loss, argued that life is not merely lived; it is spoken, misheard, deferred. He famously stated that the

DOI: 10.4324/9781003728764-2

unconscious is structured like a language,[8] emphasising that human desire emerges not from instinct, but from the entry into language. The moment the infant enters the symbolic order (the big Other as the realm of language and culture) it loses the unity of the Imaginary and becomes a split subject (*'sujet barré'*).[9] This loss inaugurates the subject's struggle: not for literal life, but for subjective coherence in the face of alienation. We are stitched into being by the signifier, fractured by desire.

Slavoj Žižek adds that we do not merely struggle in reality, but in fantasy – fantasy being the stage upon which (the noumenal of) the Real appears, clothed, bearable.[10] It is not that we suffer illusions, but rather that illusions are precisely the texture of our being.[11] Classically Freudian: like the dream, their 'purpose' is to protect us from waking up.[12] Lacan's son-in-law and editor of his Seminars, Jacques-Alain Miller, emphasises the ethical dimension of psychoanalysis. The task is not to normalise or adapt the subject to social norms, but to help the subject construct a singular way to live with their symptom. The struggle for life becomes the struggle for a mode of enjoyment that does not destroy the subject – a delicate negotiation of desire, language, and the Real of the body.[13]

Together, Žižek and Miller recast the Lacanian insight that to be human is to be caught in structures beyond comprehension (language, the Other, ideology), and that the struggle for life is fundamentally the struggle to subjectivise this condition. It is not about eliminating lack or achieving mastery but learning to live with the impossibility at the core of being.

Last but not least, psychiatrist and Holocaust survivor Viktor Frankl, staring into the abyss of Auschwitz, stressed that survival was not contingent on food or strength, but on meaning. Those who have a 'why' to live can bear with almost any 'how.'[14] The psyche endures not by the biology of instinct alone, but by 'humanities' like poetry, prayer, or promise.

This book explores what is most promising for humans in terms of enjoyment and the pursuit of meaning in life. Could it be as simple as feeling love and being loved? The experience of love plays a crucial role in contemporary research on happiness across psychology, neuroscience, and sociology. Studies consistently identify close, affectionate relationships as key predictors of well-being. Love is integral to authentic happiness, and relationships are considered foundational to human flourishing.[15] Longitudinal studies, such as the *Harvard Study of Adult Development*, further demonstrate that the quality of loving bonds is a more robust predictor of long-term happiness and health than wealth or career success.[16] Neuroscientific research has shown that experiences of love activate the brain's reward systems, thereby enhancing emotional regulation and fostering trust.[17] In addition to its affective benefits, love also contributes to eudaemonic well-being, offering individuals a sense of meaning, coherence, and purpose.[18] Taken together, love emerges not only as a source of pleasure but as a structural condition (not for survival but) for truly human thriving. We might argue, therefore, that more important than the struggle for life is the struggle for *love*. When properly analysed, it consists of three kinds of struggle: the struggle *for* love, the struggle *to* love, and the struggle *of* love.[19] They will appear in varying proportions throughout this book.

The Struggle for Love

Let us begin with the struggle *for* love. A mouth before a mind, a cry before a word: the infant reaches not only for milk but for being. In the arms of the primordial Other (usually the mother), we encounter the first rhythms of love: warmth, presence, and responsiveness. But inevitably, instead of mirrors, we meet fractures. Thus begins a lifelong struggle for love, marked by a yearning for something lost before it could be named. From a psychoanalytic standpoint, this struggle originates in infancy, rooted in the earliest attachments. Freud viewed love as emerging from the dynamics of the libido: the infant's desire for the mother serves as the prototype for all subsequent longing.[20] Early experiences of gratification and frustration lay the groundwork for how love and desire are pursued throughout life. They serve as templates for subsequent relationships, with persistent echoes of unmet needs and unconscious repetitions.

Moreover, love is never just affection; it is knotted with need, lack, and fantasy. It is never free of the unconscious. We are drawn to objects of love that resemble caregivers who withheld affection or were unable to be pleased. This repetition compulsion reflects a drive to resolve unhealed wounds, but it also exposes the anxiety at the core of love: Do I deserve love? Will I lose it? The pursuit of love is haunted by the spectre of abandonment and the hope of redemption. Freud suggested that the libido moves from object to object, attaching, detaching, and reattaching – like bees around flowers – never fully satisfied. Love becomes a search for the lost original object.[21]

Lacan deepens this sense of longing, describing us as subjects of lack, split by language, forever alienated from the Real.[22] The beloved becomes a screen for the projections of early desire. 'I love you,' says the unconscious, 'but only if you love me in the way my mother never did.'

In this light, love is not merely about affection or companionship but an ontological pursuit, a longing to be seen, recognised, confirmed: *Tell me I exist.* But the Other is not our mirror. They are a subject in their own right, not a saviour. Love, chased as salvation, often arrives as misrecognition. What we find is never quite what we hoped for, because it is always filtered through the unconscious past. Lacan's theory of the mirror stage clarifies this dynamic. When the infant first recognises its image in the mirror, it misrecognises wholeness in a fragmented body, producing what Lacan terms *méconnaissance*.[23] This foundational alienation introduces a structural lack into the subject's being. The Other (whether caregiver or future lover) becomes a placeholder for an imagined completeness that was never truly possessed. Love thus becomes a fantasy of return to that illusory unity, a striving to recover what was lost with the break from the maternal body. Love is less about the actual qualities of the Other than about the fantasy they carry. As Lacan famously puts it, love is giving something you don't have to someone who doesn't want it.[24] This paradox captures the impossibility and the excess woven into the desire for love. Because the Other is always already embedded in language and desire, love becomes a demand: one that inevitably surpasses what the Other can offer. It is a call for recognition that exceeds the bounds of what recognition can satisfy.

Relational psychoanalyst Jessica Benjamin reframes this by emphasising that love is also a quest for mutual recognition.[25] The subject seeks to be affirmed by the Other, not as a mere reflection, but as an autonomous self. Love thus becomes a space where the need for validation and ontological security meets the burden of psychic history. After all, romantic love is often overloaded with unconscious demands, expected to heal the scars of early neglect or abandonment.

For Nietzsche, the fundamental force animating life was not the will to survive, but the Will to Power – a creative, dynamic striving to overcome, to assert, to transform oneself and the world.[26] In this light, the struggle for love can be viewed as a sublimated form of this will to power: not domination in the crude sense, but a longing to affirm one's existence in the eyes of the Other, to shape the self through desire, and to find transcendence in the vulnerable act of giving and receiving love. Love, like art or philosophy, becomes an arena for the expression of one's singular intensity: a site where *becoming* is at stake. Marx, by contrast, situates struggle in the material and historical world of class conflict.[27] Love does not float above society; it is embedded in the relations of production, shaped by ideology, and stratified by inequality. The struggle for love is also a struggle within capitalism's commodification of intimacy, in which human relations risk becoming transactional, alienated, or subordinated to economic logic. Where Nietzsche's Will to Power elevates love to a creative force of individuation, Marx's class struggle reminds us that love unfolds on terrain that is already contested and unjust. Between these poles (the existential and the political), psychoanalysis maps the middle ground: the unconscious theatre where power and desire intertwine, and where the fight for recognition, dignity, and psychic coherence plays out.

Ultimately, the struggle for love is a struggle for being. It is mediated by lack, driven by fantasy, and animated by repetition. In seeking the Other, we are seeking ourselves *through* this Other, but never entirely *in* them.

The Struggle to Love

If the struggle *for* love is the plea to be loved, the struggle *to* love is the more daunting task: to love the Other *as* Other, beyond the projections of one's needs, fantasies, and fears. It requires a movement beyond the mirror, beyond the self-reflection that seeks confirmation rather than connection. Erich Fromm famously asserted that love is not a passive emotion but an active art.[28] It demands patience, discipline, humility, courage, and a capacity for inner freedom. To love is not simply to fall, but to *stand* in love, again and again. It is an ongoing practice, rather than a fleeting feeling.

From the outset, love is entangled with ambivalence. Melanie Klein demonstrated how the infant both loves and hates the breast, cherishing it for nourishment while resenting its absence.[29] This ambivalence becomes structural: to love is also to tolerate frustration, to accept the beloved's failure to complete us, and to love still. Klein's concept of the depressive position encapsulates this achievement: the psychic capacity to hold love and hate together and relate to the other as a whole object, rather than as split into idealised or persecutory parts. True love does not eliminate aggression; it integrates it. As Freud and later theorists observed, Eros always dances with Thanatos.[30] Even when love flourishes, it is shadowed by destructive impulses. The beloved is both sanctuary and storm – an object we wish to preserve, but may also wish to harm, precisely because they matter so much.

Donald Winnicott adds another essential dimension: the ability to love presupposes a stable enough *true self* and a *good-enough* early environment.[31] The caregiver must allow frustration and separation within a secure holding context. Mature love, then, is the capacity to be alone together, i.e. to preserve psychic separateness while remaining emotionally connected.[32] Fusion may tempt us, but symbiosis forecloses the other's subjectivity. Early object relations shape our capacity to love. If early caregivers were intrusive, absent, or inconsistent, love may feel unsafe. Defences such as withdrawal, idealisation, clinging, or aggression may arise, not as flaws, but as remnants of earlier attempts at psychic survival. The struggle to love thus involves dismantling these outdated protections to make room for intimacy.

A core psychoanalytic insight is that we often love not the actual other but what the other represents in the unconscious. Idealisation can mask narcissistic investments; the beloved becomes a mirror of our own wish for wholeness. True love, by contrast, demands de-idealisation. It asks us to recognise the beloved not as an extension of ourselves, but as a subject with their own desire, history, and opacity. This is where love meets its limits and matures.

Lacan sharpens this existential tension: 'Love is giving something you don't have to someone who doesn't want it.'[33] Love is not the fulfilment of needs but an encounter with lack. We offer our absence, our incompletion, and are met in return by the other's own unfilled void. Love is not a bridge over lack, but a dialogue through it.

Even when love is found and returned, it does not resolve. It stirs, destabilises, and seethes. It opens old wounds (the absent father, the engulfing mother, the formative silences) and reactivates their traces. Yet, in this very destabilisation lies its potential for transformation. Love is a paradox: it soothes and stings, heals and haunts. Thus, the struggle *to* love is not a failure but a process. It is a developmental and ethical achievement: an ongoing negotiation among desire and recognition, fantasy and reality, and self and other. It requires psychic flexibility: to move between symbiosis and separation, to withstand ambivalence, to remain open to the other without annihilating difference. Where the struggle for love seeks to be seen, the struggle to love dares to see. To *make* love is to recognise the Other in their irreducible alterity. It is probably the most intimate and most difficult act (of love) of all.

The Struggle of Love

Love, even when found and given, does not rest. It seethes. It shifts. It stumbles. The struggle *of* love is the struggle of paradox. It addresses contradictions *intrinsic* to love. As Freud noted, love lives with its shadow, hate.[34] Eros and Thanatos dance in every kiss. We desire and resent, cling to and push away the same person. We wish to preserve the object of our love, and sometimes, to destroy it, precisely because it matters too much. *I hate to love you!*

Following Lacan, we give the void; we offer lack. And in return, we are offered another's absence. Love is not a bridge over this lack. It is a dialogue through it. Moreover, he argues that desire is always the desire of the Other, that is, it is formed in relation to the Other's desire, never purely autonomous.[35] Thus, even in love, we are caught in a web of misrecognitions and unconscious repetitions. The more we demand from the Other what only a lost object could give, the more we find ourselves frustrated.

Even when attained and reciprocated, love does not grant peace. It awakens longings and anxieties that destabilise the self. Love misfires because no amount of love can fill the subject's existential void. The Oedipal complex dramatises this: the child loves the parent but also competes with them. The beloved becomes both sanctuary and threat, saviour and rival.

The child's love for the parent is often overlaid with feelings of rivalry, jealousy, and guilt. These unresolved dynamics resurface in adult relationships, often reenacted through transference. Romantic love becomes a theatre in which early conflicts are revived under the illusion of newness.

Finally, love often oscillates between desire and domestication. Desire thrives on absence, mystery, the unreachable. But love seeks presence, security, familiarity. In long-term relationships, this creates a tension: Can desire survive stability? Can eroticism coexist with emotional safety? It is the struggle with time. Love may begin with idealisation, a fantasy of fusion, but reality imposes limits. Long-term love requires the endurance of disillusionment. As Winnicott notes, the ability to tolerate the Other's failure to attune to us perfectly is foundational to the emergence of mature object relations.[36] The other changes, or we do. We project unmet needs, recreating childhood scenarios in adult relationships. Even in mutual love, the unconscious persists. It acts out old traumas, resurrects infantile fears. Thus, the struggle of love is also the struggle to maintain it in the face of real-life challenges, unconscious sabotage, and the limits of human understanding. In love, this means allowing space for the real person to emerge, even when they contradict our fantasies. Love, in this mature form, is less about fulfilment than about mutual recognition and the capacity to repair.

Lacanian theory further deepens the paradox of love. Desire, according to Lacan, is always the desire of the Other,[37] meaning that love is never purely spontaneous or authentic; it is structured by the unconscious and the symbolic field. Furthermore, the tension between desire and demand means that love is often caught between the wish to be recognised and the impossibility of being fully understood.

The Logics of Love

The proverb says that all is fair in love and war. Both follow their own peculiar logic. For the French philosopher André Comte-Sponville, love lies beyond morality.[38] When we act kindly towards our loved ones or those dear to us, we do not do so out of ethical conviction but simply out of love. For this philosopher, morality is a *'semblant'*/semblance of love. Since not everyone is dear to us, and we cannot love everyone, we behave morally when we treat others *as if* we love them. Something similar applies to the relationship between ethics and etiquette. Politeness is likewise a semblance of morality. When we say '*pardon,*' '*excuse me,*' or '*sorry,*' it is *as if* we feel guilty. When we say '*please,*' it seems we genuinely care about the other person's well-being. In other words, we act *as if* we treat the other with moral concern.

According to the French philosopher Luc Ferry, we are living through a revolution of love. In the past, we may have been willing to die for God, country, or other ideals.[39] Today, only love remains as something for which we would be willing to sacrifice our lives. Love is the last remaining sacred value; *sacred* in the sense of something we hold dear above all else. Allow me to put it poetically:

Love, the gold that still survives,
The last to glow when nothing thrives,
A light that lives where darkness drives.

But there are many forms of love. In our popular culture, romantic love takes centre stage. It is this love that most often features in pop songs. It is typically characterised (put somewhat clinically) by a pleasant feeling of emotional attraction towards a person, often (but not always) accompanied by an erotic component. There is a deep and powerful desire to connect with an idealised beloved, with the hope that such feelings will lead to a shared future. Idealisation forms the core of romantic love, but it also underlies the bond between parents and children. When all goes well, babies and their parents are, for a time, each other's most beautiful and beloved beings on earth.

Love is a complex emotion, composed of elements of passion and attachment, which may or may not coexist. Passionate love involves excitement and activates the brain's pleasure centres with a dopamine release akin to that triggered by cocaine.[40] According to neuroscientists, this state typically lasts only 12 to 18 months.[41] Attachment love, on the other hand, is characterised by calmness and safety. Social psychologists understand love as a fusion of passionate love (accompanying physical arousal), intimacy (a feeling of closeness), and commitment (an investment in and effort towards the relationship).[42]

Historically, the term 'romantic' derives from medieval chivalric romances. Romantic love in this early sense was popularised by the ideal of *courtly love,* celebrated by the troubadours. This courtly love is a curious invention whose traces can still be discerned in contemporary rituals of courtship. It is love conceived as purified perfection, as pure refinement, as a form of art. Religious motifs associated with the Virgin Mary also contributed to the image of a noble lady who is attentively and chivalrously wooed, and this aristocratic ideal has left an enduring mark on our experience of love. Here we encounter a culture – even a cult – of love that, in a kind of alchemy, is sublimated into a higher, more elevated form. It is one of many examples of how culture and ideology, operating largely outside our awareness and therefore with an almost natural ease, shape our behaviour, our experience, and even our most intimate attachments. In some regions, snails and insects are considered delicacies; in others, the mere thought of eating them provokes disgust. What we find 'tasty' is determined by culture not only on our plates, but also between the sheets – and again in ways that appear entirely 'natural.'

Biologically, love takes shape through the formative force of parental care, the healing power of social and communal bonds, and the romantic love whose unmistakable hormonal dimension, expressed through copulation and reproduction, is essential to species survival. In the two temporalities of attraction and attachment, the latter may develop into an emotional bond with someone missed in their absence, with whom, rhythmically or not, sensory stimuli are exchanged, more or less mutually desired. In a one-liner: love is fiction and sex is friction.

Many neurobiologists point to the links between love and the neural pathways of desire, feeding, and addiction. Maternal love is universal in higher animals. Winning or keeping the beloved is considered by biologists to be one of the strongest motivators of behaviour. Sexuality is something quite different: it may occur without any bond or attachment whatsoever – and, conversely, attachment may exist without sex. Among mammals, there is nonetheless a clear overlap, as the 'love hormones' oxytocin and vasopressin play a role in both phenomena, which may help 'explain' the close connection between love and lust.[43] Neuroimaging studies have shown that romantic love and parental love are distinct yet overlap.[44] Both involve a reduction of critical evaluative functions, which immediately accounts for the typical blindness of lovers.

Love has many faces, and not all of them are gentle. It can also be obsessive, anxious, or even violent. When love turns into addiction, jealousy, or hatred, its destructive side comes to the fore. Some psychoanalysts claim that every love carries within it a seed of madness. This is perhaps most evident in the tragic love stories that fill our literature, from *Romeo and Juliet* to *Les Liaisons Dangereuses*. In clinical practice, the connection between love and suffering is familiar. Many patients consult a therapist because they cannot bear the pain of love: its absence, its loss, its distortion, or its impossibility. Love has a healing power. Winnicott emphasised that, in good-enough parenting, a child receives a loving, containing presence that enables the development of a true self.[45] The analytic setting, too, may function as a loving space: a place where the unloved parts of the self are met with understanding and care. Such therapeutic love is not erotic, nor sentimental, but steadfast and transformative.

Speaking of Love

For more than a century of (nowadays worldwide) listening to people talking uncensored about their erotic and love life, psychoanalysis has learned a lot about its vices and vicissitudes. In psychoanalytic practice, the ground rule of free association remains valid to this day. The patient is encouraged to speak out and thus say things he would not tell anyone else, not even to himself! As a result, he regularly jumps (not logically but associatively) from one thought to another. Fragments of truth can appear from this 'draft.' Trying to forge them neatly into a conclusive whole would rather serve the fabrication of a lie, and any theory produced along the way is at best a fruitful mistake. In this regard, I refer to the short-story writer Barthelme: 'Fragments are the only forms I trust.'[46] Isn't the language of desire fragmentary? It breaks through existing frameworks and keeps thinking in motion.

Along these lines, I consider essays an appropriate format for a revealing blend of poetic evocation and scientific thought. In doing so, the pudding of the brain can enter into treaties with the chops of the heart. At best, essays combine the playful with the lucid and thus characterise themselves by *ludicity*.[47] Michel de Montaigne said of his *Essais*: '*C'est moi que je peins*.'[48] What I paint is myself. The essay reports on a thought that, above all, is searching and finds itself therein. Doesn't this also fit the description of the psychoanalytic enterprise, where, after all, musing and thinking are mainly done out loud? The stirrings of our souls remain half-cooked; only in the mouth are they formed. Dixit *Dada-poète* Tristan Tzara: *La pensée se fait dans la bouche*.[49] Or in the pen, of course!

A kaleidoscope fractures the vision of a single object or scene into a multitude of different but interrelated forms of the same. The book's multiple perspectives render it kaleidoscopic. The essays that follow draw on a wide variety of scientific, philosophical, cultural, and psychoanalytical sources. While covering a wide range, they each stand entirely on their own. They can therefore be read in one go or piece by piece. It is mainly the lovely subject matter, the psychoanalytical perspective and my voice that ought to warrant their coherence.

Notes

1 Darwin, C. (1859). *On the origin of species by means of natural selection*. London: John Murray.
2 Hobbes, T. (1651/1996). *Leviathan* (R. Tuck, Ed., p. 88). Cambridge: Cambridge University Press.
3 Camus, A. (1942/1991). *The myth of Sisyphus* (J. O'Brien, Trans.). New York: Vintage International.
4 Freud, S. (1920). *Beyond the pleasure principle* (J. Strachey, Trans.). New York: Norton. Cave: because I publish in both Dutch and English, I sometimes refer to the English version and sometimes to the Dutch or original version of Freud's and Lacan's work.
5 Freud, S. (1923). *The ego and the id* (J. Strachey, Trans.). New York: Norton.
6 Bowlby, J. (1969). *Attachment and loss: Vol. 1. Attachment*. New York: Basic Books.
7 Schore, A. N. (2003). *Affect dysregulation and disorders of the self*. New York: Norton.

8 Lacan, J. (1966). *Écrits* (p. 500). Paris: Seuil. Structured *like* a language as *a system of difference*. I stress the word 'like' rather than 'as.' Also, language should not be reduced to the verbal. See, for example, Dall'Aglio, J. (2025). What sort of language is the unconscious structured like? A Lacanian neuropsychoanalytic perspective. *The Psychoanalytic Quarterly*. https://doi.org/10.1080/00332828.2025.2565998. Every response of the (m)Other is symbolic/digital (and not only imaginary/analogous) from the very beginning. In that sense, the infant is thrown into Lacan's signifiers as a 'signifying chain.' Freud's Id is an energetic field, and some signifiers bind/'pacify' better than others. I referred to the image of the Liquid Crystal Display with us, subjects, at the interface of energy and signifier in Kinet, M. (2023). *The spirit of the drive in neuropsychoanalysis*. London/New York: Routledge.

9 Lacan, J. (1966). *Écrits* (p. 819). Paris: Seuil.

10 Žižek, S. (2006). *How to read Lacan*. New York: Norton.

11 Žižek, S. (1989). *The sublime object of ideology*. New York: Verso.

12 Freud, S. (1900). *The interpretation of dreams. Standard edition* (Vol. 5, pp. 339–627). London. Hogarth Press.

13 Miller, J.-A. (2011). The unconscious and the speaking body. *The Lacanian Review*, *1*, 11–20.

14 Frankl, V. E. (1946/2006). Man's search for meaning (I. Lasch, Trans., p. 76). Boston: Beacon Press.

15 Seligman, M. E. P. (2002). *Authentic happiness: Using the new positive psychology to realise your potential for lasting fulfilment*. New York: Free Press.

16 Waldinger, R. J., & Schulz, M. S. (2010). What's love got to do with it? Social functioning, perceived health, and daily happiness in married octogenarians. *Psychology and Aging*, *25*(2), 422–431.

17 Zeki, S. (2007). The neurobiology of love. *FEBS Letters*, *581*(14), 2575–2579.

18 Ryff, C. D. (1989). Happiness is everything, or is it? Explorations on the meaning of psychological well-being. *Journal of Personality and Social Psychology*, *57*(6), 1069–1081.

19 Struggle for, to and of are – of course – abstract/ideal types. These were introduced by sociologist Max Weber as the one-sided accentuation of one or more points of view and the synthesis of a great many diffuse, discrete, more or less present (and occasionally even absent) concrete individual phenomena. Weber, M. (1922/1949). *The methodology of the social sciences* (E. A. Shils & H. A. Finch, Trans.). New York: Free Press.

20 Freud, S. (1905/1953). Three essays on the theory of sexuality (J. Strachey, Trans.). In J. Strachey (Ed.), *The standard edition of the complete psychological works of Sigmund Freud* (Vol. 7, pp. 123–243). London: Hogarth Press.

21 Freud, S. (1905/1953). Three essays on the theory of sexuality (J. Strachey, Trans.). In J. Strachey (Ed.), *The standard edition of the complete psychological works of Sigmund Freud* (Vol. 7, pp. 123–243). London: Hogarth Press.

22 Lacan, J. (1949/2006). The mirror stage as formative of the function of the I. In *Écrits: The first complete edition in English* (B. Fink, Trans., pp. 75–81). New York: Norton.

23 Lacan, J. (1949/2006). The mirror stage as formative of the function of the I. In *Écrits: The first complete edition in English* (B. Fink, Trans., pp. 75–81). New York: Norton.

24 Lacan, J. (1972–1973/1999). *The seminar of Jacques Lacan, Book XX: Encore, On feminine sexuality, the limits of love and knowledge* (B. Fink, Trans., p. 263). New York: Norton.

25 Benjamin, J. (1988). *The bonds of love: Psychoanalysis, feminism, and the problem of domination*. New York: Pantheon.

26 Nietzsche, F. (1911/1967). *The will to power* (W. Kaufmann & R. J. Hollingdale, Trans.). New York: Vintage Books.

27 Marx, K., & Engels, F. (1848/1992). *The communist manifesto* (D. McLellan, Ed.). London: Oxford University Press.
28 Fromm, E. (1956). *The art of loving*. New York: Harper & Row.
29 Klein, M. (1946/1997). *Envy and gratitude and other works, 1946–1963*. New York: Vintage.
30 Freud, S. (1920/1955). Beyond the pleasure principle (J. Strachey, Trans.). In J. Strachey (Ed.), *The standard edition of the complete psychological works of Sigmund Freud* (Vol. 18, pp. 1–64). London: Hogarth Press.
31 Winnicott, D. W. (1960). The theory of the parent-infant relationship. *International Journal of Psycho-Analysis*, *41*, 585–595.
32 Winnicott, D. W. (1958). The capacity to be alone. *International Journal of Psychoanalysis*, *39*, 416–420.
33 Lacan, J. (1972–1973/1999). *The seminar of Jacques Lacan, Book XX: Encore, On feminine sexuality, the limits of love and knowledge* (B. Fink, Trans., p. 263). New York: Norton.
34 Freud, S. (1915/1957). Instincts and their vicissitudes. In J. Strachey (Ed. & Trans.), *The standard edition of the complete psychological works of Sigmund Freud* (pp. 117–140). London: Hogarth Press.
35 Lacan, J. (1958). The direction of the treatment and the principles of its power. In: *Écrits: The first complete edition in English* (B. Fink, Trans., pp. 489–542). New York: Norton.
36 Winnicott, D. W. (1953). Transitional objects and transitional phenomena. *International Journal of Psychoanalysis*, *34*, 89–97.
37 '*le désir, c'est le désir de l'Autre*' in Lacan, J. (1966). *Subversion du sujet et dialectique du désir. Écrits* (pp. 793–827). Paris: Seuil.
38 Comte-Sponville, A. (1995). *Petit traité des grandes vertus*. Paris: PUF.
39 Ferry, L. (2010). *La Révolution de l'amour. Pour une spiritualité laïque*. Paris: Plon.
40 Fisher, H. E. (2004). *Why we love: The nature and chemistry of romantic love*. London: Henry Holt and Company.
41 Zeki, S., & Romaya, J. P. (2008). The neurobiology of love. *FEBS Letters*, *582*(14), 2577–2584.
42 Sternberg, R. J., & Weis, K. D. (2006). *The new psychology of love*. New Haven, CT: Yale University Press.
43 Young, L. J., Catania, C. A., & Wang, Z. (2005). Hormonal influences on the neural circuits underlying behavior: Oxytocin and vasopressin. *Current Opinion in Neurobiology*, *15*(6), 690–698.
44 Bartels, A., & Zeki, S. (2000). The neural basis of romantic love. *NeuroReport*, *11*(17), 3829–3834.
45 Winnicott, D. W. (1960). Ego distortion in terms of true and false self. In *The maturational processes and the facilitating environment* (pp. 140–152). London: Hogarth Press.
46 Barthelme, D. (1981). *Sixty stories*. New York: Putman.
47 De Cauter, L. (2007). De oorsprong van het spel. In N. Vliegen & L. Van Lier (Red.), *Een spel voor twee spelers. Spel en speelsheid in de psychoanalytische therapie*. Leuven-Leusden: Acco.
48 de Montaigne, M. (1580/1979). *Essais*. Paris: Flammarion.
49 Tzara, T. (1924/1978). *Sept manifestes Dada. Lampisteries*. Paris: Fayard.

3

Love's Infinitives

What Do We Talk About?

Some 3000 years ago, the poetess Sappho of Lesbos claimed that love causes pain and spins fairy tales.[1] To this day, no subject has received more attention or inspired more words than love. God may have been declared dead, but love remains vibrantly alive. For some, simply speaking about love is a pleasure in itself.[2] Yet, the question posed by Raymond Carver ('What do we talk about when we talk about love?') is by no means easy to answer.[3] There are many types of love: romantic love, altruistic love, parental love, platonic friendship, but also love of country, love of cycling, or (as in this book) love of psychoanalysis. Love is not only a value in and of itself; it is also a value that imparts meaning and worth to other things. Moreover, love differs for each person and in every moment. It is both universally human and singular. It is a universal trait that every experience of love is perceived as unique. This does not preclude the possibility of uncovering certain truths about love; truths that, to varying degrees, shape its forms and trajectories.

Greek Love

From a philosophical perspective, thinkers since Antiquity have distinguished three main types of love: *eros*, *philia*, and *agapē*.[4] In the Greek tradition, *eros* (like Freud's libido) is broader and more expansive than mere adult sexual desire. It encompasses the full range of human longing that transcends basic needs, which concern only self-preservation.[5] *Eros* is primarily the love driven by desire, by a sense of lack. It is love as *I want you*. It is also the kind of love discussed by the Athenians in Plato's *Symposium*.[6] Aristophanes recounts the myth of the spherical, double-backed creature that was split in two by Zeus for its arrogance and *hubris*. Ever since, we have been searching for the lost unity with our other half. In our personal prehistory, this may refer to the close bond we once had with our (*matrixial*) mother. Torn from her, we are cast into the world. We remain infused with a yearning to return to that lost paradise. The result is the romantic ideal of the One True Love with whom everything is supposed to 'click' – happily ever after.

DOI: 10.4324/9781003728764-3

Of course, everyday reality quickly relegates that vision to the realm of fairy tales. These beautiful songs never last, and sooner or later, a new 'one true love' appears. Hence, the Lacanian slogan: '*Il n'y a pas de rapport sexuel.*'[7] Something is always amiss: a lack or absence. We will later see how this is connected to the (Lacanian) notion of 'castration.'

Eros is physical, powerful, and intense, and it can lead to a loss of (self-)control. It pierces us with its arrows or sets us alight with its torch. Sexuality is *hot stuff.* When Freud's *Rat Man* first experiences the pleasure of sexual intercourse, he exclaims: 'But this is wonderful! You could kill your father for this!'[8] *Eros* is thus the kind of love of which the poet says: One year of fire, 30 years of ash. Or more prosaically: this kind of love is like soup – the first spoonfuls are too hot, the last too cold.

Philia, by contrast, is much gentler. It is the (friendly) love that finds joy in, takes pleasure from. In Spinoza's typically abstract definition, it is joy caused by an external source.[9] Already in his *Ethics*, Aristotle wrote extensively about this form of friendship, distinguishing between various levels.[10] Some friendships are based on sensual pleasure. These only last as long as they remain 'pleasant' and are thus fleeting and superficial. Others are grounded in utility: what benefit does the relationship provide? Such bonds dissolve once they are no longer useful. Only the third type of friendship – complete or '*theleia' philia* – is true friendship, and it is a rare good. This *philia* means, simply put, taking delight in the other and genuinely caring about their well-being.[11] This marks an important distinction from *eros*, which does not necessarily benefit the beloved. Passionate love can even run counter to one's own best interest.

Philia is, by definition, happy love. The ancient Greeks valued it above all other forms because it occurs between people who view one another as equals. While *philia* does not contain a sexual element, its intimacy has the power to transform *eros* from physical lust into a more spiritual bond. Perhaps that is why Aristotle characterises marriage as a relationship grounded in *philia.*[12] In a classical or early Freudian view, the sexual drive in *philia* is goal-inhibited and sublimated. Due to the Oedipus complex, love is stripped of its sensual component and (at least consciously) only its tender flow remains.[13] Yet, in contemporary psychoanalysis, the focus has shifted to attachment, which plays a more pivotal role. It endures through joy and sorrow, in good times and in bad. Generally, *philia* tends to outlast *eros*. Every love is a transference (of) love, and every love object is a rediscovered one. Thus, *eros* and *philia* are transferred onto later figures who (consciously or unconsciously) remind us of our first loves.

Agapē originates in Paul's letters to the Corinthians and in the thought of thinkers such as Thomas Aquinas.[14] It is a selfless, altruistic, and generous form of love that extends to every person in the world, regardless of rank, status, expectation, or judgment. As such, it forms the hard and mysterious core of Christianity. It is a sacred love, for it is far from self-evident: Love thy neighbour as thyself. As though loving oneself were a given!

A Psychoanalytic Primer

In contrast to a philosophical approach, psychoanalysis is distinguished by its focus on the (early) childhood roots of love.[15] For many, this makes things seem more complicated than they need to be. For the sake of clarity, then, a brief introductory interlude is in order. At first, Freud saw love primarily in relation to our infantile sexuality. It is a pleasurable economy that inevitably unfolds in response to mother, father, and other intimate figures. It is implicitly and explicitly shaped by the prevailing laws, rules, and norms, and it bears the mark of very concrete (both pleasant and unpleasant) experiences that, whether we like it or not, set the tone for our later love life.

'Forgotten' (and thus unconscious, for where else would forgotten things reside?) desires and the associated conflicts are transferred onto whom and how we love later in life.[16] In every beloved, we partly see a reflection of ourselves, and the jubilant, idealising fascination so characteristic of falling in love always contains a fundamentally narcissistic dimension.[17] Significant encounters also always contain a dimension of recognition – a re-encounter with figures whose imprints have settled deep within our psyche. Love, moreover, never appears in its pure form. There is always a blend of positive and negative emotions, and the extent to which we can tolerate this ambivalence and ambiguity determines both the depth and durability of our relationships.[18]

Freud's (psycho-)logic was rather patriarchal. Among the Anglo-Saxon post-Freudians, the emphasis shifted more towards the mother-child relationship. For them, it is not the father but the mother who plays the leading role. To quote Otto Rank: *'Im Gegenteil, die Mutter!*/On the contrary, ze mozer!'[19]

Melanie Klein was the first to further elaborate on this early childhood dynamic.[20] She added to Freud's final drive theory – with its struggle between *Eros* and *Thanatos*, life and death drives – an object relations theory that shifted the focus of inner development to the fate of self- and object-representations populating the psyche. Through her invention of play therapy, she discovered two positions from which we perceive the world.

In the first (schizoid-paranoid) position, a preliminary ordering emerges from chaos: day and night, presence and absence, good and evil, love and hate. These opposites are split and kept apart to ward off fears of annihilation.[21] Only in a later (so-called depressive) position do we come to realise that both the inner and outer worlds contain positive *and* negative aspects. What's more, 'evil' is found not only in the other but within us as well. This gives rise to empathy and remorse. Instead of punishing or destroying ourselves, we develop a desire to repair and make amends for the harm we may have caused.[22] Through this process, love becomes more realistic and mature: complexity can now be expressed rather than repressed or split off. The internalisation of our love objects gives us a sense of emotional goodness and stability – a foundation that supports our capacity to love with greater confidence and security.

Donald Winnicott emphasised the importance of a *holding and facilitating* maternal environment for the emergence of a true and authentic self.[23] He focused in particular on the child's transition – made possible by the mother – from a sense of omnipotence to the recognition that the world and the other exist independently of one's own wishes. His famous transitional objects (e.g. a teddy bear, a blanket) facilitate this shift and serve as building blocks for play, creativity, and culture.[24]

Wilfred Bion added a third fundamental element, in addition to love (L) and hate (H), namely knowledge (*K*). *L* enables the processing and integration of experiences.[25] *H* obstructs or destroys connections and meanings. *K* is characterised by an open and receptive attitude towards new experiences and is crucial to the psychoanalytic process.[26]

Building on attachment theory, Peter Fonagy emphasises that therapeutic progress depends above all on a caring relationship that does not abandon the subject. For genuine improvement, true concern is a necessary condition that allows insight to become effective.[27]

A markedly different figure, of course, is Jacques Lacan, with his distinctive emphasis on the subject, on (specifically human, symbolic) language, and on the lack or absence inherently associated with it. The subject, for Lacan, is something entirely different from the ego, which mistakenly believes itself to be the master of its own house. The ego, in his view, is a trap – a false mirror image – for man is, echoing Sartre, not full *of* being; he is no *être*, but *néant* – a void.[28] He is an emptiness that must endlessly constitute itself through a symbolic order that logically precedes him.[29] The final word is never said, and therefore, the subject must continue to speak. The lack of being and the impossibility of full articulation together keep the engine of desire running.

Applied to love, Lacan proposes that it is a matter of giving what one lacks.[30] One gives the other a lack, a gap – and in doing so, a dynamic of mutual love is created. Falling in love belongs to the imaginary register, in which the other appears to fill the lack. One is, as it were, 'in love' with the image of the other. *Love*, by contrast, requires recognising this lack and accepting the vulnerability and dependency it entails. All of these elements point to a central insight: psychoanalysis requires no God to understand love. In a somewhat cynical aphorism, love is composed of sex and a mirror and is above all a female invention, in particular, an invention of the mother. According to Winnicott, every ordinary devoted mother is, at the moment of her child's birth, in a state of grace.[31] She gives all she has, 24/7, to her completely dependent and helpless infant. Without her, we cannot live; without her, we cannot be. She creates space for spontaneity, vitality, and creativity, and she grants us, at the right moments, the illusion that we can perform magic. Her love is initially unconditional. Even when we turn against her with hostility, she continues to offer us her cheek.

Moreover (in a Cartesian paraphrase), it is not I who thinks, but *she* thinks me: *Elle pense, donc je suis*.[32] Only if and when this mother sees us (with love) as feeling and thinking beings, can this dormant potential take root and blossom within us. Like the poet and his muse, we henceforth form with her an inner *thinking and dreaming couple*, on which we may draw again and again in moments of need.[33]

In truth, every mother bears something of the Virgin Mary within her. She is holy without effort. If we were fortunate, we fell into the proverbial butter as children and seem to draw lifelong magical strength from it. We owe this to an *abundantia cordis*: a Sacred Heart with which we identify, and which underlies later acts of generosity.

Everyday Love

Now that we have primed the canvas with some philosophical and psychoanalytic groundwork, we turn to how love manifests itself in daily life. In common parlance, love is often equated with (if not reduced to) romantic love, with all its implicit or explicit erotic dimensions. The image of romantic love is strikingly uniform. First and foremost, it appears involuntary, uncontrollable. The lover has no choice. There is a feeling, a pounding heart, butterflies fluttering in the stomach, or a body seized by other irresistible forces. Reason is squeezed into too-tight shoes, and the danger of losing one's head looms large.

Romantic love seems inevitable and, to varying degrees, tends to generate anxiety and tension, hand-wringing, and sleepless nights. We can rally every available defence to resist or guard ourselves against this love, or we can simply go with the flow. One of its essential characteristics is that it presents itself as a force of nature: one that imposes itself upon us, even sweeps us away or floods us. Curiously, we simultaneously long for and fear being delivered over to its imperatives. The danger lies in a total loss of self. Love is, in truth, a mystery to us and, as is often the case, we seek the key to that mystery *outside* ourselves.

Whether we have been struck by lightning, pierced by Cupid's arrows, or infected by a virus ('Falling in love is like catching a cold; there's nothing you can do about it, and it passes on its own'), in all cases the cause is located beyond us. Romantic love is born of chance, accident, or misrecognition. It cannot be forced or commanded and is, in any case, never the product of the will.

Love presupposes freedom. But what then of marital duty, for example? To address this, we must consult quite different conceptions of love – those summed up by the title of a widely read and long-standing bestseller by my compatriot Alfons Van Steenwegen: *Love is a Verb*.[34] The core message is that love requires effort and commitment. This, of course, refers to a love that lasts longer than *9½ Weeks*.[35] It is love with a rougher grain, the kind that endures after difference and disagreement, when the dream of unity must make way for a non-dreamt reality.

It is love in its more mundane, prosaic guise, where intimacy increasingly becomes *in-team-acy*, and cohabitation evolves into co-habituation. The team, as the saying goes, stands for Together Each Achieves More, for instance, in areas of (re)production and (pro)creation. After the pleasures of seduction and lovemaking come the burdens of procreation and cooperation. From 'all is bliss' to 'all for the kids.' This is the toll demanded by the orgy of the species. Evolutionary logic expects little more from us than that we reach maturity in order to reproduce successfully.

According to the philosopher, marriage is the lifelong exclusive ownership of each other's genitalia.[36] And according to the poet, partners in a deep and happy love eventually become the 'tender guardians' of each other's solitude.[37] Such formulations evoke a markedly different image from that of two figures embracing beneath palm trees along the water's edge. Yet, the idyllic, idealised image of love remains a deeply ingrained human *idée fixe*. It is a rose-tinted mirage that dominates, above all, the world of pulp and kitsch. Unlike art, these domains acknowledge neither division nor conflict. Good and evil are caricatured and easily distinguished, and intelligence is signalled by little more than the presence of horn-rimmed glasses.

Belief and Art

In love, we must set reason aside to make room for belief. Love begins where knowledge ends, or more poignantly: love is the panic of reason. Most people believe that not only religion but love as well should remain far removed from rationality. Love is a form of faith. Faith in a gesture, in a face: a belief that the other harbours a hidden treasure that fits our own like a lid on a pot. Love is the triumph of hope over (self-)knowledge. When it comes to both love and faith, 'using your head' is almost considered a form of sacrilege. It is as if we fear that a rational investigation would dry up the very wellsprings of belief and love alike. This view contains a kernel of truth. Love and belief are essentially products of the imagination; they are imaginary.[38] They are not encountered; they are made. A certain kind of blindness or illusion is constitutive of these experiences. When someone points out that we've fallen for the 'wrong' person, the response by Woody Allen's character in *Manhattan* is hilariously illustrative: 'I know. My psychoanalyst warned me, but you were so beautiful that I got another psychoanalyst.' This line earns our immediate sympathy. After all, hasn't the love of truth already stolen enough miracles? Hasn't science already disenchanted the world enough?

Erich Fromm speaks of *The Art of Loving*.[39] According to him, we must become aware that love (like life itself) is an art. One does not become a good musician or visual artist without sufficient knowledge and practice. Only once both have been mastered can intuition (as a synthesis of the two) take over and become the essence of every form of art. Last but not least, a striving for mastery must be the primary driving force behind it all.

Fromm criticises the fact that, in our society, nearly everything is taken seriously except love. For success, prestige, money, or power, we spare no expense or effort. But in matters of love, everything is expected to happen spontaneously. And yet, our capacity to deal with love (to experience it or to enjoy it) can grow and deepen. Of course, this kind of knowledge or skill is always limited and relative. The truth is violated when we try to capture it too rigidly. The circle never fully closes; the final word is never spoken.

Our thinking, in the words of post-Freudian Wilfred Bion, must remain 'unsaturated,' so that new meanings and perspectives may continually enter and transform it.[40]

As Socrates once said: Is the unexamined life even worth living? Two millennia before Hannah Arendt's *The Banality of Evil*, he held that there is but one good: knowledge, and that all evil stems, in one way or another, from ignorance. Does the same not apply to a good as precious as love?

How to Write (on) Love?

Another question arises: in what language should we speak of love? Inspired in part by Heidegger's *The Origin of the Work of Art*, we might distinguish between the truth-telling of science and that of art.[41] Academic language is dry; it aims for precision and unambiguity. Through a high level of abstraction, it aspires to produce universally valid (*nomothetic*) statements. Its ideal is the language of mathematics, in which (according to Galileo Galilei) the book of nature is written. Science thus seeks to capture the concrete multiplicity of phenomena in the abstract unity of a formula or theory. $E = mc^2$ or Newton's law that gravity diminishes with the square of the distance are typical examples. Art, by contrast, operates in the opposite direction. It expresses the concrete many through the $n = 1$ of the concrete singular. According to Kant, no fixed rule can be prescribed for art. Paradoxically, great art is both utterly original and exemplary. It begins in the concrete and ends in the concrete. Its statements are *ideographic*. In its own way, art also transmits knowledge – but only in the form of a unique and irreplaceable example. *Madame Bovary* is, in truth, a study of hysteria; the secret annexe of Anne Frank makes the impact of the Holocaust palpable; Magritte's *Ceci n'est pas une pipe/La Trahison des Images*[42] functions as an icon of the unknowable *Ding an sich*.

Scientists and artists are both tinkerers. In their creativity, intuition, imagination, and ordering logic are entirely intertwined. In scientific publications, the intuitive phase is always omitted. At best, it surfaces much later – in the autobiography of the scholar. For instance, August Kekulé von Stradonitz reported that he first envisioned the benzene ring structure in a dream in which a snake bit its own tail (the ouroboros). Einstein likewise recounted that his dreams were important to the development of the special theory of relativity.[43] Scientific publication proceeds rationally from question through reasoning to answer, even though in practice, the answer intuited often precedes the formulation of the question.

Everything begins with the spark; then follows a phase of uncertainty; only afterwards comes the order of publication. Anyone who has ever devised something themselves knows this to be true. In contrast to the analytical methodology of Western science, other cultures have long recognised an associative science of the concrete. Claude Lévi-Strauss refers to this as *bricolage*.[44] For him, it is not a developmental stage but a style. Moreover, Lévi-Strauss notes a major misconception about science: in every laboratory, the tradition is first to tinker, then to rationalise formally – first dream, then reality. According to the French poet René Char, the scientist searches for '*preuves*' (proofs) while the artist seeks '*traces*.' He also says that scientists define things, whereas artists 'infinitise' them (*l'infini est de définir la chose*).[45] This marks the difference between poetry and logic – or, in psychoanalytic terms, between hysteria and paranoia: the former reveals the Thing, while the latter seeks to enclose it within a totalising theoretical system. No wonder, then, that some poets (my famous compatriot Hugo Claus, for example) considered themselves incapable of rational thought altogether.[46]

A Peculiar Science

For Freud, psychoanalysis is not only a method of treatment and a science of the unconscious, but also a method of investigation. After over a century of closely listening to the fantasies, dreams, nightmares (the inner stirrings) of countless patients, psychoanalysis is undoubtedly one of the richest sources of knowledge about human (and especially romantic) life. Freud famously divided this life into two central capacities: the ability to love and the ability to work.[47] One might add *fight* to the list, for a good life often requires either combat or surrender. A mobile phone provider recently updated the triad to *Work, Love, and Play*.

The analysand's free associations and the analyst's evenly hovering attention together lead, as Thomas Ogden writes, to 'conversations at the frontier of dreaming.'[48] And is this threshold between dream and reality not, above all, the natural habitat of love? Love is mute, and what gives it voice is poetry. Love is, above all, the terrain of poets and writers, of singers and filmmakers, who praise it in their songs and illuminations. Yet, certain regularities can also be discerned in love. As Polonius remarks in *Hamlet*: 'Though this be madness, yet there is method in't.'[49] In psychic (as opposed to natural) causality, these patterns are highly particular rather than universal. Influenza produces the same symptoms in everyone, everywhere, but Mrs X's fear of fast elevators only manifests in the presence of bearded men…[50]

Psychoanalysis is the science of the irrational. Lacan even calls it the 'science of the particular' (*la science du particulier*).[51] It aims to reveal the irreducibly singular relationship of the subject to lack and loss, to the things of life, and to the discourse and desire of the Big Other – that is, the micro- and macro-culture that governs how we eat, dress, love, die, and so on. It is precisely through case studies (of which psychoanalysis has countless) that the universal emerges in the particular. In this shared focus on singularity, essay, and psychoanalysis converge. The devil (or the unconscious/demonic) is, after all, in the details.

Many scientific writings about love are, perhaps, somewhat sterile. Through their language, love is stripped of its excess and its madness. Yet, love (beyond its few animal components) is above all a profoundly human achievement. It is universal sublimation and creation, the triumph of subjectivity and imagination. As Michel Foucault put it: *la folie est absence d'œuvre* – madness is the absence of a body of work.[52] In that case, let us declare love the *chef-d'œuvre* of madness: a delirious and masterful body of work. It is at once symptom and artefact; a makeshift construction and a work of art. Love is a well-known illustration of the fact that one needs a great deal of imagination to live in reality…

Notes

1 Sappho in: Stassijns, K., & Van Strijtem, I. (2001) *3000 jaar wereldpoëzie in 500 onsterfelijke gedichten.* Amsterdam/Tielt: Atlas/Lannoo.
2 Lacan, J. (1972–1973/1998). *The seminar of Jacques Lacan, book XX, encore: On feminine sexuality, the limits of love and knowledge* (J. A. Miller, Ed. & B. Fink, Trans., p. 83) New York: Norton.
3 Carver, R. (1981). *What we talk about when we talk about love.* New York: Picador.
4 Nussbaum, M. C. (1986). *The fragility of goodness: Luck and ethics in Greek tragedy and philosophy.* Cambridge: Cambridge University Press.
5 Lacan, J. (1932/1980). *De la psychose paranoïaque dans ses rapports avec la personnalité.* Paris: Seuil.
6 Decorte, J. (Red.) (2000). *De uitgelezen Plato.* Amsterdam-Tielt: Boom-Lannoo.
7 Badiou, A., & Cassin, B. (2010). *Il n'y a pas de rapport sexuel. Deux leçons sur «L'Etourdit» de Lacan.* Paris: Fayard.
8 Gay, P. (1989). *Sigmund Freud. Zijn leven en werk* (p. 247). Baarn: Tirion.
9 de Spinoza, B. (2022). *Ethica: In geometrische trant uiteengezet* (H. Krop, Vert.). Boom, Deel III, Stelling 13, Scholium. Amsterdam. Boom.
10 Aristoteles. (1999). *Ethica.* Groningen: Historische Uitgeverij.
11 Aristoteles. (2004). *Retorica.* Groningen: Historische Uitgeverij 1380b35.
12 Aristoteles. (1999). *Ethica.* Groningen: Historische Uitgeverij 1161a en 1162a15.
13 Freud, S. (1921). Group psychology and the analysis of the ego. In *Freud standard edition* (pp. 111–112). London: Hogarth.
14 Thomas Aquinas. (1265–1274/1947). *Summa theologiae* (Fathers of the English Dominican Province, Trans.). Benziger Bros. New York, NY.
15 Bergmann, M. S. (1988). Freud's three theories of love in the light of later developments. *Journal of the American Psychoanalytic Association, 36*(3), 668 e.v.
16 Freud, S. (1905). *Drie verhandelingen over de theorie van de seksualiteit.* K.B.**1**. Sigmund Freud Nederlandse Editie (pp. 49–177). Amsterdam/Meppel: Boom.
17 Freud, S. (1914). *Over de geschiedenis van de psychoanalytische beweging.* P.B. **1**. Sigmund Freud Nederlandse Editie (pp. 59–132). Amsterdam/Meppel: Boom.
18 Freud, S. (1916). Rouw en melancholie. *Freud Werken, 7*, 129–148.
19 Gay, P. (1989). *Sigmund Freud. Zijn leven en werk.* Baarn: Tirion.
20 Kinet, M. (1996). Weerzien met…Melanie Klein. *Tijdschrift voor Psychotherapie, 22*, 197–211.
21 Klein, M. (1952/1975). The origins of transference. In *The writings of Melanie Klein. (Vol IV)*. London: Hogarth Press.
22 Klein, M. (1935/1975). A contribution to the psychogenesis of manic-depressive states. In *The writings of Melanie Klein* (Vol I). London: Hogarth Press.
23 Winnicott, D. W. (1960/1990). Theory of the parent-infant relationship. In *The maturational process and the facilitating environment.* London: Karnac Books.
24 Winnicott, D. W. (1951/1992). Transitional objects and transitional phenomena. In *Through paediatrics to psycho-analysis.* London: Karnac.
25 Bion, W. R. (1962/1984). *Learning from experience.* London: Karnac.
26 Bion, W. R. (1965). *Transformations.* London: Heinemann.
27 Fonagy, P. (1991). Thinking about thinking: Some clinical and theoretical considerations in the treatment of a borderline patient. *International Journal of Psychoanalysis, 72*(4), 639 656.
28 Sartre, J. P. (1943/1976). *L'être et le néant. Essai d'ontologie phénoménologique.* Paris: Gallimard.
29 Lacan, J. (1964/1973). *Le Séminaire. Livre XI. Les quatre concepts fondamentaux de la psychanalyse.* Texte établi par J. A. Miller. Paris: Du Seuil.

30 Lacan, J. (1957–1958/1998). *Le Séminaire Livre V. Les formations de l'inconscient.* Texte établi par J. A. Miller. Paris: Du Seuil.
31 Winnicott, D. W. (1949/1950). The ordinary devoted mother and her baby. In *Nine broadcast talks.* London: Pamphlet.
32 Cluckers, G., & Meurs, P. (2005). Bruggen tussen denk-wijzen. In M. Kinet & R. Vermote (Red.), *Mentalisatie.* Antwerpen/Apeldoorn: Garant.
33 Grotstein, J. (1981). Who is the dreamer who dreams the dream and who is the dreamer who understands it? In J. Grotstein (Ed.), *Do I dare disturb the universe*? London: Karnac.
34 Van Steenwegen, A. (1988). *Liefde is een werkwoord.* Tielt: Lannoo.
35 Lyne, A. (Director). (1986). *9½ Weeks* [Film]. Metro-Goldwyn-Mayer.
36 Kant, I. (1797/2004). *De metafysica van de zeden* (J. Stolker & Y. Eskens, Vert., p. 147). Amsterdam: Boom.
37 Rilke, R. M. (1929/2000). *Brieven aan een jonge dichter* (P. Verstegen, Vert., p. 58). Amsterdam: Athenaeum-Polak & Van Gennep.
38 De Martelaere, P. (1994). *Een verlangen naar ontroostbaarheid.* Amsterdam: Meulenhoff.
39 Fromm, E. (1956/1995). *The art of loving* (Classics of personal development). *Re-issue Edition.* London: Thorsons.
40 Bion, W. R. (1970/1986). *Attention and interpretation.* London: Karnac.
41 Heidegger, M. (1935–1936). *De oorsprong van het kunstwerk.* Amsterdam: Boom Esthetica.
42 Magritte, R. (1929). *La trahison des images [Ceci n'est pas une pipe] [Painting].* Los Angeles: Los Angeles County Museum of Art.
43 Rocke, A. J. (2015). It began with a daydream: The 150th anniversary of the Kekulé benzene structure. *Angewandte Chemie International Edition, 54*(1), 46–50. Koestler, A. (1964). *The act of creation.* London: Hutchinson (in part III The Logic of Discovery, pp. 116–118; 144–146).
44 Lévi-Strauss, C. (1962). *La Pensée Sauvage.* Paris: Plon.
45 Char, R. (1950). Les matinaux. In *Œuvres complètes.* Paris: Gallimard, coll. Bibliothèque de la Pléiade, 1983.
46 Claus, H. (2004). *Groepsportret. Een leven in citaten* (p. 84). Amsterdam: Bezige Bij.
47 Freud, S. (1916–1917). Introductory lectures. In *Freud standard edition* (Vols. 15–16, p. 457). London. Hogarth Press.
48 Ogden, T. (2002). *Conversations at the frontier of dreaming.* London: Karnac.
49 Shakespeare, W. (1603/2006). *Hamlet* (A. Thompson & N. Taylor, Eds.). London: Arden Shakespeare, Act 2, Scene 2.
50 Green, A. (1995). *La causalité psychique. Entre nature et culture.* Paris: Odile Jacob.
51 Lacan, J. (1972–1973/1975). *Le Séminaire Livre XX. Encore.* Texte établi par J. A. Miller. Paris: Du Seuil, Leçon 8/05/1973.
52 Foucault, M. (1961). *Histoire de la folie à l'âge classique.* Paris: Gallimard.

4

Lovestruck

A False Truth

Somewhere in *Beyond Good and Evil*, Nietzsche remarks that a false judgement is just as important as a true one: 'to give up false judgements would be to give up life itself.'[1] A well-known statement by Aleksandr Pushkin echoes the same sentiment: the illusion that moves us is dearer than ten thousand truths.[2] Anyone who has ever experienced the seven delights of being in love will immediately and wholeheartedly affirm the utterances of these two nineteenth-century gentlemen. In the enamoured state, one would much rather be mistaken and in love than uncertain and loveless. To outsiders, lovers may seem utterly deranged. Yet, they convincingly string together a chain of illuminated moments. Like blind seers, they see only what truly matters. They may be in every state imaginable, yet they can also state everything.[3]

Freud compares falling in love to a state of hypnosis, a practice he soon abandoned, incidentally, because he found it cosmetic: it concealed problems rather than resolving them.[4] In his study, *Group Psychology and the Analysis of the Ego*, Freud elaborates on the idea that, within a crowd, individuals identify horizontally with one another.[5] Differences between them are effaced in a regressive movement, and the crowd becomes a primitive, many-headed monster. There is a vertical identification: the leader becomes the common ideal, a *Führer* or *Duce*. This is a form of idealisation in which a particular object is invested with all power and/or libido. This kind of idealisation is not only a group psychological phenomenon but also an individual psychological one. It is operative in hypnosis and in romantic love, where the object appears perfect. In its extreme form, Freud argues, this may lead to amorous servitude: the lover becomes a kind of serf to their idealised object.

In psychoanalytic literature, falling in love has been likened to a *foule à deux* (a crowd of two), to a *folie à deux*, and also to a *narcissisme à deux*.[6] It can equally be viewed as a revival of the divine mother-and-child dyad. In a forward flight, it was precisely this coupling that once saved us from our helplessness and disarray. Do we not always fall for someone who seems whole while we ourselves feel fragmented and confused? And is there any form of love more intense than that

DOI: 10.4324/9781003728764-4

between mother and child? How else can we describe their mutual rapture and their 'I only have eyes for you, baby'? How often does the outside world try in vain to share in their joy – a joy from which it ultimately feels excluded? Or else, how often do disbelieving bystanders simply and 'objectively' wonder what all the fuss is about?

The Mirror

Jacques Lacan introduced the mirror stage into developmental psychology.[7] It is the moment when the human infant – still physiologically immature and barely holding itself together – jubilantly (mis)recognises itself in the mirror. This mirror should be understood both literally and figuratively. The child reflects itself not only in the glass but, more significantly, in the eyes of the Big Other. Strictly speaking, what occurs is not a recognition but a (narcissistic) identification, one that is linguistically marked and/or mediated by a third party. The child identifies with a (mirror) image and simultaneously becomes alienated from itself. A distinctive feature of Lacanian psychoanalysis is its insistence on the illusory status of the ego, understood not as an agency but as a specular one.

We dwell on the mirror stage because it is crucial for understanding how falling in love installs the imaginary order. In love, this imaginary register reaches its zenith. It clarifies why, alongside love and adoration, a (latent) element of hatred is often active in infatuation. The gap between the devaluation of the self and the idealisation of the object – between smallness and grandeur – and the accompanying sensation of dependency necessarily implies an aggressive component for the lover. *I hate how important you are to me.* In the post-Freudian theories of Melanie Klein, this aggression acquires mythical proportions and is conceptualised as a constitutional envy or death drive.[8] Lacan sees it as inextricably linked to the mirror stage. In connection with love, he therefore proposes the neologism *hainamoration* (from *haine*, hatred, and *amour*, love): a cocktail of hate, love, and admiration.[9]

Newborns

Existentialists say that love rescues us from our '*Geworfenheit*' or thrownness.[10] The romantic fatalism in which lovers believe they were made or born for one another has its roots in experiences from the neonatal period. We are reminded of a remark by Victor Hugo: *'Qu'est-ce que des amants? Ce sont des nouveau-nés'*[11] (lovers are like newborns). We are especially susceptible to falling in love during times of separation, abandonment, or existential need. In summary, we might say that love is the sum of an inner necessity and an act of imagination. According to Freud, our helplessness creates a lifelong need for love. These mechanisms manifest in extreme ways in the Stockholm syndrome, in which a hostage feels vitally dependent on their captor and subsequently develops feelings of sympathy, or even love.[12]

We often say that falling in love is something that happens to us, that overtakes us. It is something bodily, something non-verbal – or rather, preverbal: a glance, a touch, something in a voice that catches our attention. A magnetic pull is activated through which we lose ourselves and dissolve into another, with whom we now wish to unite – completely and exclusively. These are moments in which we become almost speechless, utterly spellbound by an enchantment we neither can nor dare to break. Silence takes the floor. Or the sea. Or the stars. Lovers flee into each other's arms, removing themselves from both the social order and any form of comparison. In doing so, they reinvent the warm water of love for the umpteenth time. The unique feeling that accompanies this amorous adventure is, strangely, one of its most universal features. Curiously, this whole upheaval arises precisely through a kind of ignorance. In love, it seems, unfamiliarity breeds affection rather than contempt. We fall in love when we do *not* know each other – and we feel wounded when we do.

At First Sight

Love at first sight takes the crown in this respect. In this context, Lacan even speaks of an algebraic unknown: the small a object (*objet petit a*) that we suddenly believe we have found (or rather, *re-found*) in the other. *Re-found*, because for psychoanalysis, as well as for Kierkegaard's love at first sight for his muse Regina, it is essentially a matter of *recollection*.[13] This *objet petit a* is like a bubble or a 'flaw' in the field of perception, through which the Thing reveals itself. The seemingly 'natural' sexual attraction or excitement turns out, on closer inspection, to contain an intricately layered network of profound and complex meanings. In those few nanoseconds – those microdots – of erotic magnetism or, more broadly, of love at first sight, an entire unconscious psychosexuality is condensed.[14] You recognise *something in* someone because you have always already known them. In the words of psychoanalyst Adam Phillips, the beloved contains something both familiar and alien. He calls it a 'familiar foreign body.'[15]

According to Colette Soler, the *coup de foudre* marks a moment in which the Big Other of language is short-circuited, opening a direct passage to the drive.[16] This drive is only ever partially socialised or symbolised, and its *jouissance* may suddenly erupt in the form of intense arousal or release. In such moments, we are entirely at the mercy of the drive – overtaken by it, helpless before it – even when the experience feels utterly 'wrong' for all sorts of reasons. The way *jouissance* can surface abruptly is both unsettling and destabilising; it does not belong to the neat and familiar order of ordinary experience. One might think, for instance, of an involuntary bodily response to an unexpected stimulus in a public space, or of the confusing mixture of tenderness and excitation that may appear in a situation of proximity between generations.

A Rosy Psychosis

Unlike passion (which may be regarded as its runaway variant), being in love is an inspiring condition. We are filled with the presence of the other, to whom we wish to surrender ourselves with Dionysian fervour and enthusiasm. Freud describes how, in love, the distinction between *I* and *Thou* dissolves, and an oceanic feeling arises: 'a pure pleasure-ego confronting a strange, threatening external world.'[17] Various objects become fetishised: displaced symbols and erotic substitutes for the beloved. A paperclip, a hairpin, a lighter, or the armrest against which a head once rested can each evolve into a sensual relic of the absent one.

Falling in love also brings about a surge of libido. This libido is largely withdrawn from the multitude of other loved 'objects' and from the self in which it had been distributed. Instead, all libido becomes concentrated in one dazzling apparition. There is both a bodily and a spiritual idealisation of the object, which distinguishes love from mere desire. Temporarily, a range of inhibitions and repressions can be lifted, allowing sexuality to transgress its habitual boundaries – even those approaching the perverse. This may lead to more experimental or playful forms of intimacy, in which the partners explore the full range of bodily and emotional contact. Naturally, all this can also be read in terms of the early infantile, oral-narcissistic symbiosis in which lovers temporarily form a self-contained Whole-All.

The idealisation inherent in love ultimately lifts the subject above the everyday, elementary economic logic of the pleasure principle. We would move heaven and earth for a single glance from our beloved, spare no effort or expense, just to hear their voice on the telephone for a moment. Every separation or absence is wholly coloured by waiting and longing, by the lacerating texture of lack. For the lover, the beloved is the all-good mother from our deepest dreams – one who gives us everything and denies us nothing.

Is love, according to psychoanalysis, no more than a rosy psychosis? And even if it is, so what? According to Freud, we must be neurotic enough to strive for goodness with integrity, perverse enough to be able to enjoy, and psychotic enough to transform reality. He famously quipped that those who never lose their minds over something have no mind to lose.[18] This state of being in love is, in any case, finite and therefore (without cynicism) has a favourable prognosis. It exists by virtue of misrecognition and illusion, in which lovers still appear to each other as a filling of one another's lack. Sometimes, this enamoured state can give way to love. And it is only in that state that difference ceases to make a difference.

Angles

Marriage may be good, but it is never delightful, said La Rochefoucauld.[19] The comfort marriage provides is meagre, for it belongs to a different, non-imaginary order. It has to do, among other things, with honesty, which, supposedly, lasts longer. For marriage, falling in love is not a dream but a threat or a nightmare. Or it may be an escape from the hinterlands of the everyday. Jane Austen calls these 'a quick succession of busy nothings.'[20]

In a cartoon by my compatriot Kamagurka, set in Suburbia, we see, on the one hand, an illuminated, noisy bedroom window suggesting a couple in full swing. Outside the house, a suspiciously bouncing car is parked, containing another shadowy, rocking pair. Caption: 'After thirty years of marriage, Gerda and Karel finally climaxed together.' Once again, according to La Rochefoucauld, the chains of marriage are sometimes so heavy that it takes three people to carry them. This marks the beginning of a fatal trigonometry teeming with algebraic unknowns, in which straight lines give way to angles and curves. Psychoanalysis interprets such sexual adventures as a return to our childhood. It was then that we witnessed the *première* of this (Oedipal) drama of passion. It unfolded so turbulently that we repressed it. But not to worry: it will resurface later (in fresh and ever-changing guises) in our adult relationships.

Notes

1 Nietzsche, F. (1886/1993). *Voorbij goed en kwaad.* Amsterdam: Arbeiderspers.
2 Pushkin, A. (1825/1977). *Scene from Faust.* In W. H. Bruford & H. W. T. Heath (Eds. & Trans.), *The prose tales of Alexander Pushkin* (pp. 229–231). London: Oxford University Press.
3 Moyaert, P. (1994). *Ethiek en sublimatie. Over de ethiek van de psychoanalyse van Jacques Lacan.* Nijmegen: SUN.
4 Freud, S. (1921). *Massapsychologie en Ik-analyse.* C.R.**5**. Sigmund Freud Nederlandse Editie (pp. 11–93). Amsterdam/Meppel: Boom.
5 Freud, S. (1921). *Massapsychologie en Ik-analyse.* C.R.**5**. Sigmund Freud Nederlandse Editie (pp. 11–93). Amsterdam/Meppel: Boom.
6 Green, A. (2002). *La Pensée clinique.* Paris: Éditions Odile Jacob.
7 Lacan, J. (1949). Le stade du miroir comme formateur de la fonction du Je. In *Ecrits* (pp. 93–100). Paris: Du Seuil.
8 Klein, M. (1957/1975). Envy and gratitude. In *The writings of Melanie Klein* (Vol. IV). London: Hogarth Press.
9 Lacan, J. (1991). *Le Séminaire. Livre VIII. Le transfert.* Texte établi par Jacques-Alain Miller. Paris: Seuil.
10 Heidegger, M. (1927/1962). *Being and time* (J. Macquarrie & E. Robinson, Trans.). New York: Harper & Row.
11 Hugo, V. (1862/2008). *Les Misérables.* Paris: Gallimard.
12 Namnyak, M., Tufton, N., Szekely, R., Toal, M., Worboys, S., & Sampson, E. L. (2008). "Stockholm syndrome": Psychiatric diagnosis or urban myth? *Acta Psychiatrica Scandinavica, 117*(1), 4–11.
13 Lowrie, W. (1970). *Kierkegaard* (Vol. 1, p. 202). Gloucester: Peter Smith.
14 Stoller, R. (1979/1986). *Sexual excitement: Dynamics of erotic life* (p. 165 e.v.). London: Karnac.
15 Phillips, A. (2012). *Missing out: In praise of the unlived life* (pp. 37–38). London: Penguin.
16 Soler, C. (2009). *What Lacan Said about women: A psychoanalytic study.* London: Routledge.
17 Freud, S. (1930). *Het onbehagen in de cultuur.* C.R. **3**. Sigmund Freud Nederlandse Editie (pp. 79–173). Amsterdam/Meppel: Boom.
18 Lessing, G. (1772/2012). *Emilia Galotti.* London: Emereo.
19 De La Rochefoucauld. (1665). *Maximen - bespiegelingen over menselijk gedrag,* vert. Maarten van Buuren. Groningen: Historische Uitgeverij, 2008 maxime 113.
20 Austen, J. (1814/2016). *Mansfield park.* London: Pan McMillan.

5

First Love

Rewind

When people speak of their first love, they usually refer to their adolescent years rather than their early childhood. Yet, we seem to have forgotten that this was an extremely passionate time, marked by intense emotions, daily dramas, and a fair share of sex and violence. What romances and conflicts played out in the playground? And what clandestine or sexual activities occurred behind the scenes? Psychoanalytically, we assume that even before these recallable romantic adventures, earlier enactments have occurred. Never spoken aloud by any of those involved, these were played out through interactions – relational patterns that inscribed blueprints into our psyche, decisively shaping many later experiences. Most familiar are the scenarios of the Oedipal period. We cannot recount the script, but we enacted the desire to be the darling number one of one parental figure, and by extension, to eliminate all rivals. When we triumphed, we felt like royalty; when we lost, we were left to wonder: Who is that other person I am not, and what does that person have that I lack? Lacanians call this elusive 'something' the phallus: supposedly what fully satisfies the beloved. Fully, so that no one else can slip in a word (or a phallus) edgewise.[1]

Freud identified the prototype of all subsequent love in the child's first passionate attachments.[2] Love, as he saw it, repeats itself endlessly, returning in disguised form to its earliest objects. We fall again and again for the same *somebody else*: the one who, without knowing it, carries traces of our first caregivers. Laplanche later refined this view by describing how the adult's unconscious messages – enigmatic, seductive, and overflowing the child's comprehension – implant the seed of infantile sexuality.[3] Each smile, each tender or intrusive touch, is charged with meanings the infant cannot yet decode, and these residues later structure desire. Our first love is not a sentimental memory but a sedimented field of signifiers: gestures, voices, rhythms, and gazes that have etched themselves into our nervous system.

Infant Research

Thanks to infant research (Daniel Stern, Beatrice Beebe) and developments within neuroscience (Colwyn Trevarthen, Allan Schore), many of Freud's insights have been refined or specified. These findings also address the critical concern raised by the

DOI: 10.4324/9781003728764-5

philosopher of science Adolf Grünbaum: that psychoanalysis requires validation *outside* the consulting room to claim scientific credibility.[4] It has since become clear: not only the child (as William Wordsworth put it), but also the infant is father to the man.

Human infants begin expressing love at a very early age. The most basic bodily language of affection is learned around the fourth or fifth month of life. Striking similarities appear when comparing adult and infantile motor behaviour: gazing into each other's eyes without speaking, physical proximity (especially face-to-face), continuous bodily contact, and changes in vocal patterns. There are also many synchronous movements and specific (love-related) gestures such as kissing, hugging, touching, and holding hands or faces. From two and a half months onwards, infants can sustain mutual eye contact for up to a minute – something they do not do with other 'objects.' Adults look each other in the eyes for more than five seconds only for two reasons: to fight or to make love. In French, the phrase captures it more poetically and precisely: *ils se regardent quasi constamment*. It visually echoes Winnicott's famous statement: 'There is no such thing as a baby.'[5] There is only the inseparable dyad between the infant and the caregiver (typically the mother).

Across cultures, parents and children (and lovers) occupy different zones of proximity. A certain interpersonal distance applies between adults (varying by individual), but only infants and lovers are permitted to stand closer. When they speak, they use a private idiom. They twist everyday language with neologisms and pet names. In this 'baby talk' or *motherese*, melody outweighs lyrics; familiar words are pronounced differently. There is a specialised register of facial expression, mirroring and exaggeration, and a kind of dance unfolds, marked by symmetrical rhythms of approach and withdrawal. This dance is not merely a vertical variation on a horizontal theme. It reflects our earliest and deepest layers of connection and communication.[6]

If we listen carefully, this early duet of gazes and gestures already contains the music of later passion. The language of lovers (filled with diminutives, whispers, and playful nonsense) echoes the mother's baby talk. Schore and Trevarthen showed that these proto-dialogues sculpt the right hemisphere, the seat of affect regulation and empathy.[7] The neurobiological resonance of love thus has ancient roots: long before words, the infant learns, through synchrony, to anticipate another's rhythm and to be moved by another's emotion. The first love story is about timing.

A Tender Passion?

Controversial, of course, is the erotic nature of the Oedipal configuration. Many children express a wish to marry a parent, but do they also want to share a bed? You can love your mother or father, but do you also find them attractive? This can be inferred not only from children but also from adult recollections. The first sexual stimuli and experiences take place within the family circle and are subsequently subjected to the incest taboo. Sexual appetite gives way to repression and disgust, much like our excretions once did. No initial attraction, no taboo.

Child observations reveal that pelvic movements often express waves of affection and that even before the Oedipal phase (ages three to five), children flirt. Their love lives involve not only affection but also passion, with its characteristic bursts of arousal, dramatic crescendos, and phases of activation and relaxation. Playing these registers gives the child various thrills.[8] Were children once in love with their parents, or do they move directly into companionate love? And does romantic infatuation always require an undercurrent of sensuality: repressed, sublimated, or emerging? According to Daniel Stern, children fall in love repeatedly, while their psychosexual development ensures they fall in love differently and more deeply each time.[9] The outlines are fixed; the content evolves.

Ferenczi's idea of the *confusion of tongues* between the language of tenderness and the language of passion adds another layer.[10] When the adult's unconscious invests the child with desire, the child's affectionate gestures can become erotically charged without the child's awareness. This is not perversion but the origin of symbolic life: the displacement of sensual energy into fantasy, play, and imagination. The taboo, as Lacan would later remark, is the birthplace of desire.[11] What we cannot possess, we begin to dream.

Beyond the visible and video-recordable interactions, an essentially invisible subjectivity begins to take shape. Before the end of the first year, intersubjectivity emerges: the awareness that our experiences differ from those of others. Once this leap occurs, psychic and physical intimacy (so vital in love) becomes possible. In the transitional space that opens up, the couple experiences the wonder of word-making and world-making. This anticipates what lovers later share: a unique *colloque singulier* in which they co-create and narrate their lives.[12] The exclusive focus on a single person (the concern for their being) also finds its roots in early childhood. By the end of the first year, intimacy, safety, and attachment have narrowed to one caregiver. The child becomes acutely sensitive to the presence and absence of this unique figure. Partial permeability of the boundary between self and other, as well as reciprocal identification and imitation, are already present at this stage.

Bowlby's attachment theory and Ainsworth's empirical observations confirmed how these early bonds form enduring 'internal working models.'[13] Each later love revives the first attachment pattern: secure, avoidant, ambivalent, or disorganised. The lover's anxiety when a message goes unanswered, the compulsion to repair after quarrels, the terror of loss: all these echo the infant's primal experience of separation. 'The first love,' wrote Proust, 'is only the training for the great one that will follow—but the heart remembers its apprenticeship forever.'[14] His narrator's obsession with Swann or Albertine evokes the persistence of early templates: love as the repetition of an old wound seeking new form.

Know How

Our first love shapes not only whom we love later but also *how* we love. The peculiarities of our bodily love language, the scope and depth of our shared subjectivity, the way we form joint perspectives: all of it is stored in the sensorimotor patterns of our implicit or procedural memory.[15] Without realising it, they function like key signatures for the score of our adult relationships.

In the analytic setting, this primordial score is replayed with uncanny precision. Transference love repeats the structure of first love: fascination with an idealised other who seems to hold the key to our being.[16] The analyst, like the early caregiver, receives the patient's gaze and projected desire, oscillating between tenderness and aggression. The consulting room may become a theatre of the first passion, where the analysand re-enacts both the longing for union and the fear of engulfment. When the analyst bears this projection without seduction or withdrawal, a new experience of love (less fused, more reflective) can be born. The analytic relation thus transforms the archaic into the symbolic, allowing the patient to love again without losing themselves.

Artists, too, revisit the scene of first love. Each image of longing recalls the primal dyad: the mixture of innocence and danger that defines love's origin. From Dante's Beatrice to Proust's Odette, the beloved is always a return of the first Other, that impossible figure who once mirrored and misrecognized us. Perhaps this is why first love never dies: it was never fully lived, only enacted in gestures too small to remember and too vast to forget. The mother's face as a mirror, the father's laughter as a horizon, these fragments compose the archaeology of our affect. Each later passion excavates its traces. Neuropsychoanalysis confirms that implicit memory has no timestamp: the limbic system replays early affective scripts whenever a new beloved appears.[17] Hence, the shock of recognition we call falling in love: not discovery, but some kind of *déjà vu*. It feels as if we have known each other since time immemorial!

The psychoanalytic task, then, is not to return to the lost paradise but to recognise its traces without being trapped by them. Our first love teaches us both connection and separation, tenderness and taboo, dependence and individuation. Every subsequent love oscillates between these poles. Maturity (if it exists in love) means to know that every embrace carries the ghost of the first, and that every parting repeats the primal loss that made love possible in the first place.

Notes

1 Lacan, J. (1966/1977). *Écrits: A selection* (A. Sheridan, Trans.). New York: Norton.

2 Freud, S. (1905/1953). *Three essays on the theory of sexuality.* In J. Strachey (Ed. & Trans.), *The standard edition of the complete psychological works of Sigmund Freud* (Vol. 7, pp. 123–245). London: Hogarth Press.

3 Laplanche, J. (1999). *Essays on otherness.* London/New York: Routledge; Kinet, M. (2025). Che Vuoi ? Epiloog in enkele contrapunten. In M. Hebbrecht & J. De Vleminck (Red.), *Verleiding en vertaling. Het enigma van de seksualiteit* (pp. 173–189). Antwerpen/'s Hertogenbosch: Gompel&Svacina.

4 Grünbaum, A. (1984). *The foundations of psychoanalysis: A philosophical critique.* Berkeley: California University Press.

5 Winnicott, D. W. (1964). *The child, the family, and the outside world* (p. 88). Oxford: Penguin Books.

6 Stern, D. N. (1977). *The first relationship: Infant and mother*. Cambridge: Harvard University Press.
7 Schore, A. N. (2012). *The science of the art of psychotherapy*. New York: Norton; Trevarthen, C. (1993). *The self born in intersubjectivity: The psychology of an infant communicating*. In U. Neisser (Ed.), *The perceived self* (pp. 121–173). Cambridge: Cambridge University Press.
8 Stern, D. (1993/2018). Acting versus remembering in Transference Love and Infantile Love. In E. Person, A. Hagelin & P Fonagy (Eds.), *On Freud's 'Observations on transference-love'* (p. 97). London/New York: Routledge.
9 Stern, D. N. (1985). *The interpersonal world of the infant*. New York: Basic Books.
10 Ferenczi, S. (1933/1988). *Confusion of tongues between the adults and the child*. In M. Balint (Ed.), *Final contributions to the problems and methods of psycho-analysis* (pp. 156–167). London: Karnac.
11 Lacan, J. (1958/1998). *The seminar of Jacques Lacan, Book V: The formations of the unconscious* (J.-A. Miller, Ed.; R. Grigg, Trans.). New York: Polity.
12 Person, E. S. (1988) *Dreams of love and fateful encounters: The power of romantic passion*. New York: Norton.
13 Bowlby, J. (1988). *A secure base: Parent-child attachment and healthy human development*. New York: Basic Books; Ainsworth, M. D. S., Blehar, M. C., Waters, E., & Wall, S. (1978). *Patterns of attachment: A psychological study of the strange situation*. New York: Erlbaum.
14 Proust, M. (1927/1954). *Le temps retrouvé*. In P. Clarac & A. Ferré (Éds.), *À la recherche du temps perdu* (Tome III, pp. 897–1274). Paris: Gallimard/Pléiade. p. 1033: "Le premier amour est seulement un entraînement pour celui qui suivra. Mais le cœur se souvient toujours de son apprentissage."
15 Beebe, B., & Lachmann, F. M. (2014). *The origins of attachment: Infant research and adult treatment*. London/New York: Routledge.
16 Freud, S. (1915/1957). Observations on transference-love (Further recommendations on the technique of psycho-analysis III). In *The standard edition of the complete psychological works of Sigmund Freud* (Vol. 12, pp. 157–171). London: Hogarth Press.
17 Solms, M. (2013). *The conscious id. Neuropsychoanalysis*, *15*(1), 5–19. https://doi.org/10.1080/15294145.2013.10773711

6

Labrador Love

Yofi and Bruce

Martin (Freud's son) did not mean to criticise the British way of life when he remarked that 'a dog seems almost like the head of the household here.'[1] This is by no means a specifically British phenomenon, for his own Austrian family was equally enamoured of dogs. Sigmund Freud kept a Chinese Chow, and his daughter Anna owned a German Shepherd. Both dogs reportedly barked incessantly at every patient entering the house on the *Berggasse*, but Yofi (the chow) was so well-trained that she often attended Freud's psychoanalytic sessions. Thanks to her internal clock, her master didn't even need a watch to end consultations on time.[2]

Roy Grinker's account of his analysis with Freud is particularly revealing in this regard. On one occasion, when he became very emotional, Yofi jumped onto him, prompting Freud to remark: 'You see, Yofi is so excited that you've discovered the root of your anxiety!'[3] Yofi means 'beautiful' in Hebrew, and she apparently possessed a remarkably refined psychoanalytic sensibility. It's as if she could register a shift in the affective atmosphere, what Ferenczi would have called the 'vibrations' of the analytic field.[4] This may be charming folklore or the subtle truth of mammalian intersubjectivity, but, in my view, it is rather exceptional, especially when compared with our own (more modest) experience.

For the past few years, we ourselves have had a black Labrador at home. His name is Bruce. Not named after Springsteen, Lee, or Willis, but after Almighty. He came from a litter of eleven. We visited him in the early weeks. His mother barely ate. She tirelessly performed day-and-night shifts, self-sacrificingly feeding half of her brood at a time. She was utterly depleted. I don't know why we chose Bruce in particular. According to the breeder, he was the calmest of the litter. Which prompts us to wonder how the others turned out. Bruce, at any rate, has an impressive working pedigree. His father was once the English champion. We saw a photograph of him standing tall, his tail outstretched, gazing towards a point on the horizon as if he were on the coast of Newfoundland. Meanwhile, one of Bruce's brothers has become a respected mountain rescue dog in the Swiss Alps. That's why my wife bought Bruce a red leather collar with little white crosses. It makes him look supremely trustworthy. *Quod non*, I might add.

DOI: 10.4324/9781003728764-6

Sweetheart

Naturally, we think Bruce is the sweetest and most beautiful dog in the world. He's as aerodynamic as a gleaming bullet. Now a black angel, then a black devil, he is above all our eternal baby. Gradually, our lives became fully organised around his wet and dry needs. His passive vocabulary has grown to around fifty words. He doesn't care about semantics or grammar but instantly recognises the 'motherese' or mammalian register of sounds, tone, and timbre. When he looks back at us without words, his gaze is a form of address that precedes grammar, and he exposes all our pretensions to mastery. In that meeting of eyes (ours, heavy with meaning, his, luminous with immanence), we brush the edge of the Lacanian *real*: that register which resists symbolisation but animates it, nonetheless.[5] From a Winnicottian perspective, our dog occupies a transitional space (half inner, half outer) in which a child (and later an adult) experiments with dependence and autonomy, omnipotence and reality testing.[6]

A dog is not a blanket, nor is it a person; it is a living, responsive object that both receives and modulates our projections. Kohut would add that he often functions as a self-object: a mirror for our vitality, a quietly dependable presence that shores up cohesion when the human world frays.[7] For those whose early environments were misattuned, I guess the dog's reliable warmth can be an after-good-enough, a late transitional provision that restores the possibility of tenderness. In attachment terms, dogs can be vitally important as a secure base and a safe haven, perhaps especially for those whose human bases were inconsistent or punitive.[8]

Many say dogs resemble their owners. Like our car, he might reflect something of ourselves, or like a child, inherit his parents' narcissism. Bruce is our beloved and idealised alter ego. Moreover, he is unconditionally loving and accepting. He understands us without words and attunes himself purely through body language. He has something of the all-good mother who gives us everything and grants us everything, in both good and bad times. Sometimes he watches over us or takes care of us. Then he is a cross between a bodyguard and a guardian angel (or better: a house guardian). He certainly embodies an archaic parental image, while we feel like the royalty he wishes to please. None of this denies the alterity of animal life. He incarnates an alterity that unsettles our anthropocentrism. Jacques Derrida confesses to being 'ashamed' under the gaze of his cat, a shame born not of obscenity but of being seen by another who is neither God nor human: a simple reminder that our subjectivity is not the sole light in the room.[9]

Phylogenesis

We can also learn much from him about other aspects of our unconscious. As fellow mammals, we have shared a large portion of our brains for some 250 million years. Where we differ significantly is in the prefrontal cortex. In both volume and connectivity, it is proportionally much larger in humans. It governs inhibition, thereby making reflective thought possible and rendering us largely unaware of our actual drives. Our capacity for symbolism, theory of mind, and mental time travel is likewise a neocortical achievement. Genetically, the difference between humans and bonobos is smaller than that between Indian and African elephants.[10] Our intellectual capacities are incomparable, but they are morally neutral. Intelligence can be used for good or for harm. Our ethics can extend to what (or who) is radically different from us. Yet, no other species is as capable as we are of harming its own kind, starting with our mother nature. Fortunately, there is a term for this: the Anthropocene.

Affective neuroscientists make a clear distinction between drive and instinct. The drive is located deep in the brainstem. Pleasure and unpleasure function as its compass, by which internal, homeostatic processes are evaluated. Traditionally, the drive is seen as a measure of the psychic labour demanded by life: restoring disturbed equilibria (unpleasure) into renewed balance (pleasure). Instincts reside slightly higher, in the limbic system. These concern hardwired behavioural patterns and (emotional) response tendencies in relation to the environment. The migration of birds, the upstream swimming of salmon, and the hibernation of bears. They do not need to be learned; they are evolutionarily prewired.

Affective neuroscience sharpens this intuition. Mammals share a set of ancient emotional action systems – SEEKING, FEAR, RAGE, LUST, CARE/NURTURING, PANIC/GRIEF (closely allied to ATTACHMENT), and PLAY – rooted in midbrain and limbic circuitry and conserved by evolution. These are written in capitals because they correspond to anatomically and behaviourally distinct circuits. They are not metaphorical names but experimentally tractable networks that guide us and scaffold meaning long before the neocortex tells stories about them. Our dogs live inside these systems alongside us. Their bodies 'speak' the language of approach, avoidance, yearning, protection, rivalry, desire, sorrow, and delight: languages we also speak, sometimes too fluently for our own comfort. I will let Bruce illustrate.[11]

Bruce Exemplary

First, there is the SEEKING or WANTING system. When Bruce goes outside, he begins by exploring the surroundings, his tail enthusiastically wagging. He takes pleasure in the hunt for new stimuli or treasures. This is related to, but distinct from, the LIKING system. Sometimes he finds something that pleases him or matches his 'desires.' This brings a certain satisfaction, and from then on, he knows exactly where to go to find 'it' again.

Then there is the FEAR-AVOIDANCE system. Bruce does not need to be taught not to jump from stairs or other heights. His predecessors who dared such leaps did not survive the evolutionary process.

Next is the RAGE system: if cornered or if a predator targets him, he will bark or bite in self-defence. The enemy must be destroyed. This is a form of hot aggression, which must be distinguished from the cold, calculated aggression of a predator chasing its prey. Intermale aggression is a subtype. Bruce may nip his opponents' flanks or stand his ground with noisy bravado and loud barking – but he never means real harm, nor does he inflict it.

The ATTACHMENT system is (adaptively) vital for every mammal. In distress, it calls out for 'mum,' upon whose care its survival depends. In Bruce's early months, we didn't need a baby monitor to tend to his needs in a timely manner. When the caregiver remains absent too long, the 'infant' falls silent. This way, it conserves energy, remains close to the home environment, and avoids becoming an easy target because of its vulnerability. Nature is ingenious indeed.

The counterpart of the attachment system is the NURTURING system. Encountering life in need activates a caring and protective reflex. Much to some people's dismay, the female half of the mammalian species is evolutionarily better equipped to mobilise both of these instinctive patterns. Bruce once found a little hedgehog that had become trapped on its back among the rosebushes. Carefully, he freed it from its thorny predicament. I'm not sure whether this detracts from his masculinity.

There is also the LUST system, which drives us to reproduce and rewards us with a pleasure bonus for doing so. Bruce is, to this day, a bachelor and lives (despite his intact genitals) a chaste life. He shows little interest in his fellow canines and, during training, pays them no attention, remaining fixated on his master(s). When he comes for a cuddle, he insists on crawling (back) into the little hollow between my armpit and the sofa. And when my wife and I are affectionate with one another, he immediately wedges his nose between us (or might even bite ours off). On the door to my consultation room hangs a sign that reads: 'Attention. Dog in psychoanalysis.' I doubt that he is receptive to Freudian–Lacanian interpretations. In the veterinary world, I fear we must limit ourselves to behavioural therapy.

Finally, there is a PLAY system. All mammals have a kind of play drive. If mice miss their daily playtime, they have to make up for it the next day with an extra half-hour. Through play (which often comes with a few bruises), much is learned: about skills, limits, and social interaction. Bruce lays his front legs on the ground, lifts his hindquarters into the air while wagging his tail, and, when the time is right, invites us to enter the game (*Latin: in lusio*). To paraphrase the German writer Juli Zeh: If everything is a game, we are lost; if not, then certainly.[12]

Canine Clinic

We are far from pretending that Bruce solves the human enigma. Rather, living with him has taught us to read the mammalian palimpsest beneath our speech. When he burrows into the crook of an arm as if returning to a lost burrow, we feel the gravity of the ATTACHMENT system pulling at both of us. When he plants himself between our bodies – insisting on triangulation – we glimpse the ancient geometry of desire, that triangular scene where love, rivalry, and belonging braid themselves into a single knot. Play becomes our micro-ethics: a rule-governed exuberance in which bite-inhibition is learned, limits are discovered, and mutual joy is cultivated.

Clinically, pets enter the room even when they do not cross the threshold. Patients speak them into being: the dog who slept against their bed in childhood;

the cat who witnessed parental fights; the goldfish flushed away without ritual, inaugurating an early apprenticeship in melancholia. When a patient mourns a pet, we often meet layered grief. The loss is not 'just an animal'; it is the collapse of a transitional space, a self-object mirror gone dark, and an attachment bond whose mute fidelity had been a lifeline. One sometimes underestimates this mourning because it is not linguistic, but the work of grief (detaching libido and reinvesting it) occurs in affective registers older than speech.

We also recognise how pets can complicate transferences. The analyst's dog (heard in the distance or glimpsed on a screen) may become the rival child, the privileged patient, the guardian, or the indifferent witness. In such moments, the animal is folded into the analytic *mise-en-scène*, a third that expands the dyad into a small ecology of gazes and needs. Philosophically, the pet unsettles human exceptionalism without collapsing difference. Agamben writes of the zone between human and animal, where distinctions blur and violence often begins.[13] Our dogs are not *human.* They have their own forms of understanding, their own *Umwelten,* yet in their company we learn a civility of the drives. The paradox is instructive: by acknowledging what we share, we become more humane; by honouring what we do not share, we become less cruel.

Lessons

What, then, have we learned from Bruce? That a dog is not a prop but a partner: the ever-available 'good object' whose presence steadies us and whose absence cuts sharply. That love is not only a story the neocortex tells but also a choreography the midbrain enacts. That play is a pedagogy. That care and dependence, when lived in the small republic of a household, are not regressions but repetitions with a difference. They are returns to early forms of tenderness that do not infantilise but *re-animalise* us in the best sense: rooting our ethics in the body's ancient capacities for approach, protection, and joy. We have also learned (more than once, alas) that the dog's time is shorter than ours. Each shared year is 'dog-time,' accelerated and precious. To love a dog is to consent in advance to a grief one cannot yet bear. And still we choose it. Perhaps because, as psychoanalysis keeps reminding us, love and loss are not enemies but partners: each gives the other its depth. Grief is the price we pay for love. If mourning a pet can feel disproportionate, it is often because the loss pierces older layers of attachment, waking those preverbal memories Freud called *the shadow of the object*.[14] To write about our Labrador is also to write about love: its illusions and redemptions, its ethics, its neurobiology, and its transference.

When Bruce curls into sleep, paws twitching in the theatre of dreams, we are tempted to ask him what he sees. Panksepp tells us that PLAY and SEEKING sketch their own oneiric landscapes.[15] Freud would add that wishes (even simple, somatic, sometimes earthy) stage themselves in sleep in ways that tame and express desire.[16] We will never know Bruce's dream in our words. But we can lie near him and let the old systems hum together – his and ours, like sympathetic strings. The room grows quiet. Without speech. Only music. In a mammalian key.

Notes

1 Freud, M. (1973). Freud: My father. In H. M. Ruitenbeck (Ed.), *Freud as we knew him* (p. 379). Detroit: Wayne State University Press.

2 Beck, M. (21/12/2010). *Wall Street Journal*, Beside Freud's Couch, a Chow named Jofi; Coren, S. (2010). *The pawprints of history: Dogs and the course of human events*. New York: Free Press.

3 Grinker, R. (2001). My father's analysis with Sigmund Freud. *Annual of Psychoanalysis, 29*, 35–47.

4 Gay, P. (1988). *Freud: A life for our time*. New York: W. W. Norton; Ferenczi, S. (1932/1988). *The clinical diary of Sándor Ferenczi* (M. Balint & N. Z. Jackson, Eds.; M. Balint & N. Z. Jackson, Trans.). Cambridge: Harvard University Press.

5 Lacan, J. (1966/1977). *Écrits: A selection* (A. Sheridan, Trans.). London: Tavistock. (Original work published 1966).

6 Winnicott, D. W. (1953). Transitional objects and transitional phenomena. *International Journal of Psycho-Analysis, 34*, 89–97.

7 Kohut, H. (1971). *The analysis of the self.* New York: International Universities Press.

8 Bowlby, J. (1969/1982). *Attachment and loss: Vol. 1. Attachment* (2nd ed.). New York: Basic Books; Ainsworth, M. D. S., Blehar, M., Waters, E., & Wall, S. (1978). *Patterns of attachment*. Hillsdale: Erlbaum.

9 Derrida, J. (1997/2008). *The animal that therefore I am* (M.-L. Mallet, Ed.; D. Wills, Trans.). New York: Fordham University Press.

10 Mens-bonobo 1.3%, Indiaanse-Indische Olifant 6–7%. Fernando, P., Pfrender, M. E., Encalada, S. E., & Lande, R. (2000). Mitochondrial DNA variation, phylogeography and population structure of the Asian elephant. *Heredity, 84*, 362–372. https://doi.org/10.1046/j.1365-2540.2000.00674.x

11 Panksepp, J. (1998). *Affective neuroscience*. New York: Oxford University Press.

12 Zeh, J. (2004). *Speeldrift*. Amsterdam: Ambo/Anthos.

13 Agamben, G. (2004). *The open: Man and animal* (K. Attell, Trans.). Stanford: Stanford University Press.

14 Freud, S. (1917/1957). Mourning and melancholia. In J. Strachey (Ed. & Trans.), *The standard edition of the complete psychological works of Sigmund Freud* (Vol. 14, pp. 243–258). London: Hogarth Press.

15 Panksepp, J., & Biven, L. (2012). *The archaeology of mind.* New York: Norton.

16 Freud, S. (1900/1953). *The interpretation of dreams*. In J. Strachey (Ed. & Trans.), *Standard edition* (Vols. 4–5). London: Hogarth Press.

7

Animal Love

Contact Comfort

When a baby cries and can be soothed only by being picked up or pressed against the breast, we say in Flemish that the child has '*pakzeer*': a deep need to be held, a 'contact comfort' phenomenon that has been experimentally studied by Harry Harlow.[1] Adults can suffer from this just as much. They often feel ashamed of such needs, which are rightly or wrongly deemed 'childish.' As a result, they may defend themselves against this longing for love. In character development, reaction formation (defending against a desire by adopting its opposite) is a common defence mechanism.[2] How many Cool Hand Lukes secretly crave nest warmth and cuddling? In the words of Olivia Newton-John: *They want to get physical,* but here, *physical* is not sexual. What they crave, first and foremost, are hugs, warmth, safety, and above all, the sensation of skin against skin.

Psychoanalytic theory is situated between two poles, both typically present in clinical practice and often in conflict with one another. One pole sees human beings as primarily pleasure-seeking, driven by lust. This pleasure may appear mysterious or morbid and serves no obvious function. Why expend so much time and energy on base jumping or bungee jumping? Why train obsessively for triathlons, or compulsively collect Matchbox cars or beer mats? The answer: just for fun. *To each their own pleasure*, as the saying goes. But, as we all know, such pleasures can seriously undermine our relationships with others.

The opposite pole stresses our fundamental drive for connection. After World War II, John Bowlby pioneered attachment research with thousands of children.[3] He distinguished two separate concepts. First, there is dependency: the child's reliance on primary caretakers who meet their physiological needs. Human infants are born immature and require extensive extra-uterine care – particularly brain development – before they can function independently. Something quite different is *attachment*. This arises from figures who tune into the child's inner world and interact with it – often through play. It is to these individuals that the child becomes attached.

Attachment theory suggests a continuity between humans and animals. It appears as though there is no real leap or threshold between them. Certainly, we share

DOI: 10.4324/9781003728764-7

at least two more rudimentary forms of love: dependency or attachment, and lust. Thomas Aquinas referred to dependency as *natural love*, which also exists between a puppy and its mother.[4] In contemporary terms, it consists of ATTACHMENT and CARE. This form of love is closely tied to the need for nourishment, warmth, and (emotional) care. Although related, dependency and attachment are not identical. In everyday language, attachment can also be a matter of habit: one may feel attached to a home, a neighbourhood, or a workplace, yet hardly miss them when relocating. In any case, these are primitive forms of love. 'True' love likely requires a form of memory found only in humans: narrative or declarative memory, which can evoke recollections, experiences, or feelings simply by hearing a name, seeing an image, or thinking of a person.

Anthropodenial

Even here, we must be cautious. How does a dog or a great ape, for example, respond after years of separation when reunited with its owner or caretaker? Some psychoanalysts, such as Alfons Van Coillie, warn repeatedly against the danger of *anthropodenial*.[5] It is the opposite of anthropomorphism: not the projection of human traits onto animals, but rather the (essentially narcissistic) human tendency to deny our kinship with our animal kin.[6]

A striking article in *Nature*, drawing on 150 years of research into chimpanzee culture, firmly contradicts this denial. The importance of culture is evident in practices such as tool use, hunting strategies, nest-building, medicinal plants, courtship, and bodily contact.[7] Not only *Homo sapiens*, but also elephants, magpies, and dolphins, for instance, are capable of mirror self-recognition. Yet, it is only in the human child that this recognition provokes a distinctive fascination and jubilation. It is considered a necessary condition for the emergence of (self-)consciousness and the development of a Theory of Mind (ToM) – an awareness of the mental states of others.

This distinctly human form of (self-)consciousness, long regarded as uniquely ours, is thought – according to primatologist Frans de Waal – to develop in layers, from the dawn of time. Similarly, it evolves throughout our personal prehistory, as various levels of self-awareness emerge.[8] When it comes to both greed and selfishness, humanity certainly takes the crown. True to Darwin, neuropsychoanalysis also repeatedly stresses differences of *degree*, not of *kind*.[9] Drawing on the work of affective neuroscientist Jaak Panksepp, Mark Solms continually emphasises the continuity between humans and other mammals (and even vertebrates). Humans share seven basic emotional-instinctual systems with them, each distinguishable by neuroanatomy, physiology, and behaviour.

For Solms, the unconscious from Freud's first (topographic) model is a memory system, and it must not be confused with the *id* from Freud's second (structural) model, which is essentially a drive- and instinct-based system.[10] These two levels inevitably remain in tension. Solms points out that bodily affects (such as hunger or thirst) and sensory affects (such as disgust or surprise) rarely – if ever – cause psychopathology. Above all, it is the *emotional* affects (attachment, care, lust, fear, rage) that generate trouble. These affects are more complex, create inner conflicts, and – last but not least – concern fellow beings with whom we share society. They present us with a delicate task – one we first confront when we are least equipped to handle it: during the Oedipal phase.[11]

Smart Animals

To cite the title of a book by Frans de Waal: *Are We Smart Enough to Know How Smart Animals Are?*[12] According to Freud, the general structure of the psychic apparatus (id/ego/superego) applies not only to humans but also to higher animals whose psychic makeup resembles our own. 'Wherever there exists, as in humans, a prolonged period of childhood dependence,' he wrote, 'one may postulate the presence of a superego.'[13] Our closest animal relatives are not merely instinctively preprogrammed. According to Frans de Waal, they undergo extensive education in impulse control[14] and, like humans, use sex to deepen bonds, offer comfort, assess compatibility, or simply for pleasure.[15] With four years of breastfeeding, they are well prepared to acquire complex social skills and relational customs.[16] Three things arguably distinguish us most from the great apes: pair bonding, symbolic/digital language (which enables science, art, and religion), and a form of sexuality governed by various taboos.

Among bonobos, for instance, there is virtually no distinction between social and sexual behaviour.[17] Human sexuality, by contrast, navigates between shame and disgust, prohibition and pleasure, the risqué and the repugnant.[18] Human love is the result of sexual repression. Repression leads to heightened arousal. Upbringing and civilisation channel and restrict the sexual drive, causing it – ironically – to reach feverish intensity and to be overvalued. In the natural state of bonobo sexuality, sex is simply ordinary, not extraordinary. It is readily available and therefore less prized. There are no precious metals, no 'noble parts.' Among bonobos, there is no romantic infatuation or idealisation of the sexual partner.

Only for humans does the sexual act receive such superlative glorification. To quote Freud's Rat Man: 'It is so wonderful one would murder one's own father for it.'[19] The human being is, in the fullest sense, an artificial creature. Perhaps we construct barriers to love precisely to enhance our pleasure.

Sheep or Wolf?

According to De Waal, primates (and especially 'hominid' great apes and humans) are essentially good. He opposes the so-called 'veneer theory,' which claims that a thin layer of morality covers a fundamentally amoral human core. Scratch an altruist, and a hypocrite bleeds. This view is loosely based on the Roman adage, popularised by Thomas Hobbes: *Homo homini lupus:* man is a wolf to man.

According to the veneer theory, only through a social contract can humanity's fundamental selfishness be corrected. De Waal, by contrast, proposes a matryoshka-doll model: the old resides within the new.[20] Mutatis mutandis, within the human being lives a great ape, a mammal, a reptile, and perhaps even something saurian. This model aligns with contemporary neurobiological insights. Researchers such as Antonio Damasio, Gerald Edelman, and Joseph LeDoux have mapped the brain's structure and function from an evolutionary perspective.[21] Popular science has since familiarised the broader public with the notion of the 'triune brain,' consisting of a primitive reptilian core, a higher (and more emotional and altruistic) mammalian brain, and the specifically human neocortex – the seat of reflective consciousness.[22]

Most primatologists argue that emotional responses underlie our moral instincts. These emotions, in their view, are the building blocks of morality. Many animals display a primitive, almost visceral form of empathy known as emotional contagion. Higher, cognitive empathy – as found in most primates – assumes some level of understanding of the causes behind another's emotions. But does this more complex helping and consoling behaviour require a rudimentary theory of mind, or is an instinctive CARE system enough to explain it? That remains an open question, since these are always hypotheses based solely on what animals do. They cannot tell us their stories.

In some cases, animal observation may be biased. The human role as participant observer could, at times, create or reinforce a dimension of 'humanity'. Consider the famous superstars: the gorilla Koko, who learned a thousand signs via sign language[23]; the chimpanzee Kanzi, who acquired human language simply by being immersed – like any human child – in a bath of mother tongue[24]; and finally, the orangutan Azy, who even reached higher levels of abstraction.[25]

Are the same processes at play here as in the case of the human child who, once upon a time, was essentially a *feral infant*? Does the child only begin to think and speak if – and only if – the Big Other (usually the mother) thinks of the child as a thinking being?[26]

From birth onward, a rich, intuitive, and affective communication emerges between mother and child. Colwyn Trevarthen speaks of *proto-conversations*.[27] This non- or preverbal register of communication remains crucial into adulthood – especially between lovers. Some researchers estimate that as much as 75% of communication is nonverbal. Depending on the theoretical framework, psychoanalysis describes these early relational dynamics using terms such as mirroring, attunement, containment, or mentalisation. The Big Other attempts to attune to the child's inner world and to assign meaning to the child's needs and appeals.

Darwin and Freud

When we speak of love for animals, we inevitably find ourselves in the borderlands between Darwin and Freud. Darwin's work (literally too, considering Freud's final London residence in Maresfield Gardens) was central to Freud's field of vision. Freud often referred to the tension between the individual and the species, in which the latter's motives and interests shape the former's actions.[28] From time to time, he also ventured into phylogeny – for example, in *Totem and Taboo*, where he traced the roots of the Oedipus complex back to the primal father and his horde.[29]

Their theoretical frameworks share a fundamental kinship: both ultimately locate the key to human behaviour in sexuality. For Freud, sexuality was the libidinal economy saturating the entire psyche; for Darwin, it was the mechanism of reproduction – the endless orgy of the species. Their insights challenge not only the proud and the puritanical but also the faithful, particularly through the role they assign to chance. For Darwin, human existence is not grounded in a Platonic ideal or divine design, but in natural selection driven by the randomness of fate. Its author (according to Steven Pinker): *The Blind Watchmaker*. And Richard Rorty rightly notes that Freud's (psycho)analysis brings us to the point where we treat chance as worthy of determining our fate.[30]

Psychoanalysis and evolutionary biology or psychology are by no means mutually exclusive. It is an established fact that humans share 98% of their DNA with chimpanzees.[31] We share a common ancestor with the primates from whom we both descend. The great apes have long been known for their high intelligence: a fact easily confirmed by any visitor to the zoo. Their courtship behaviour, displays of power, and rivalry are just as deeply marked by the Imaginary register as those of humans. Not only *fight-or-flight*, but also *freezing* and *defeat* are defensive mechanisms employed by both humans and animals in the face of aggression.

Ethology

Jacques Lacan repeatedly and explicitly linked this Imaginary register to ethological findings of his time, for instance, the work of Nico Tinbergen and Konrad Lorenz.[32] And yet, animals (including primates) do not produce art, science, labour, or prayer. Nothing indicates that they are aware of the specifically human, future-perfect tense of the deathbed. Nor do they inhabit a symbolic order, such as that represented by the (Law of the) Father.

Since the beginning of the Pleistocene, our existence has played out on the African savannahs, where we lived as hunter-gatherers and nomads in groups of 50 to 100 members. Of course, this history has left its traces. But in seeking to explain much of our behaviour as 'adaptive,' evolutionary psychology sometimes degenerates into a ludicrously simplistic form of ultra-Darwinism. For our behaviour (even our choices), explanations are sought not in our parents, but in our ancestors. Yet, as Richard Dawkins clearly states at the end of *The Selfish Gene*: 'We, alone on earth, can rebel against the tyranny of the selfish replicators.'[33]

A misunderstood neo-Darwinism likely owes part of its success to its potential to provide absolution. Instead of holding our parents responsible for our suffering and shortcomings, it offers us a convenient alibi to shift the blame onto our ancestors. And yet, as Harry Mulisch ironically observes, the impotent office clerk would do better to look for the roots (and thus the resolution) of his sexual problems not in Eve, Cybele or the Sphinx, but in *la mama*.[34] Though we might gently add that he should look within himself most of all.

Distal (evolutionary/adaptive) motives, which pertain to the behaviour and psychology of the species, do not necessarily exclude proximal motives underlying individuals' everyday actions and feelings. The former refers to the instinctual, biologically encoded drives found in the Real of our chromosomes. The latter are more accurately situated in the Symbolic order. And just as there is no longer such a thing as 'pure chance' once the symbolic has been introduced into the real, so too is the natural transformed by language.

There is a denaturing of instinct – a primordial dissonance between body and subject, nature and culture – that nonetheless continues to operate in mutually entangled ways. From this vantage point, the human being is fundamentally maladapted, and an unbridgeable gap lies between person and world.

Biological or ethological data can certainly shed light on the anthropological, but they must not be taken at face value. They require interpretation. Every psychoanalyst will acknowledge that the human being is born with a particular genetic predisposition. Yet, he is also born under a certain *constellation*: the (un)conscious fantasies, expectations, dreams, and nightmares of his parents, which exert a predetermining effect every bit as powerful as chromosomes.

Moreover, due to prolonged dependency ('upbringing'), the child's temperament is 'translated' from its very first cry. It is shaped and alienated by symbolic processes of meaning-making and by the desires of the Other. Ultimately, once grown (and somewhat conscious), the subject must decide whether to be guided by a gospel of their choosing or, in a more original way, to take destiny into their own hands.

Ethics

Since 1948, the *Universal Declaration of Human Rights* has served as a foundational instrument for establishing a global legal order. Yet it remains, for now, a noble ideal. In 2012, a group of leading international scientists signed the *Cambridge Declaration on Consciousness*, acknowledging consciousness in many nonhuman species.[35] But the ethical consequences of this recognition have hardly filtered through. Humans eat animals, wear animals, imprison animals for their milk or eggs, use them as test subjects, and so on. Clearly, the taboos against murder and cannibalism do not apply to our animal kin.

In the Western world, the consumption of great apes is considered a barbaric and dubious privilege of underdeveloped cultures. When we are confronted with images of mutilated or slaughtered gorillas (as in the work of Diane Fossey), we are instantly appalled. But our love for animals is, in truth, not much more than the 'love' between animals. It is only when we see something human reflected in them that we are moved by a naïve, sentimental sympathy. Of course, this is most evident with domesticated (if not humanised) animals. In that regard, the dog is perhaps our dearest. Loyal, unconditionally affectionate, empathetic, and wordlessly understanding, it embodies our idealised conception of mother nature. Which is why the horror is so great when, say, a lovely golden retriever turns out to have attacked an innocent victim…

Emotions may well constitute the building blocks of morality. Yet, conversely, they can also give rise to erratic and unreasonable unpredictability, if not to cruel violence. Human beings possess not only feelings but also normative ideals. We are guided not solely by our emotions, but also by rules, laws, and values. Many philosophers have sought to ground loving compassion in a shared foundation. This holds true, for instance, both in Spinoza's pantheism and in Schopenhauer's Will. It is the noumenal that binds us: the recognition that the multiplicity of appearances conceals a more fundamental, shared Being. According to Kant, morality demands that we treat other human beings as ends in themselves, never merely as means to our own ends. In every ethical decision, one must, he argued, formulate a maxim and subject it to the test of the categorical imperative. The central question, then, is whether my maxim can serve as a rational principle for all. Kant was convinced that goodness is rooted primarily in reason rather than in mere desires or emotions. Let us (poetically) imagine our animal sisters and brothers had embarked on a crusade.

Did they know the how or why?
Oh no, they just drew lots — no pope in sight!
At times, they tore a man apart with joy,
Or drained a city dry.
Now and then they'd crucify a Jesus,
Or strike down prophet, prince.
They never tired. No need to hurry.
No rules to obey.

Notes

1 Harlow, H. F. (1958). The nature of love. *American Psychologist, 13*(12), 673–685. https://doi.org/10.1037/h0047884
2 Freud, S. (1908). Karakter en anale erotiek. *Freud Werken* (Vol. 6, pp. 11–19). Amsterdam: Boom.
3 Bowlby, J. (1988). *A secure base. Clinical applications of attachment theory*. London: Routledge.
4 Aquinas. (1952). *The summa theologica of Saint Thomas Aquinas* (p. 312). Chicago: Encyclopedia Britannica.
5 Van Coillie, F. (2024). Wat we kunnen leren van ethologen over seks en gender. In J. De Vleminck & M. Thys (Red.), *Queer. Een psychoanalytische queeste* (p. 216). Antwerpen/'s Hertogenbosch: Gompel & Svacina.
6 De Waal. (2016). *Zijn we slim genoeg om te weten hoe slim dieren zijn?* Amsterdam: Atlas Contact.
7 Whiten, A., et al. (1999). Cultures in chimpansees. *Nature, 399*, 682–685.
8 Stern, D. N. (1985). *The interpersonal world of the infant*. New York: Basic Books.
9 Darwin, C. (1871/1981). *The descent of man and selection in relation to sex (facsimile)* (p. 85). Princeton: Princeton University Press.
10 Solms, M. (2013). The Conscious Id. *Neuropsychoanalysis, 15*, 5–19.
11 Solms, M. (2021). *De verborgen bron. Reis naar de oorsprong van het bewustzijn*. Amsterdam: Bezige Bij.

12 De Waal, F. (2016). *Zijn we slim genoeg om te weten hoe slim dieren zijn?* Amsterdam: Atlas Contact.
13 Freud, S. (1940). Hoofdlijnen van de psychoanalyse. I.P. 1/ 2. *Sigmund Freud Nederlandse Editie* (p. 79). Amsterdam/Meppel: Boom.
14 De Waal, F. (2022). *Anders. Gender door de ogen van een primatoloog* (p. 214). Amsterdam/Antwerpen: Atlas Contact.
15 Wrangham, R., & Peterson, D. (1998). *Agressieve mannetjes. Over mensapen en de oorsprong van geweld bij de mens* (p. 198). Amsterdam: Nieuwezijds.
16 De Waal, F. (2016). *Zijn we slim genoeg om te weten hoe slim dieren zijn?* (p. 312 e.v.). Amsterdam: Atlas Contact.
17 De Waal, F. (2016). *Zijn we slim genoeg om te weten hoe slim dieren zijn?* (pp. 295–296). Amsterdam: Atlas Contact.
18 Van Coillie, F. (2022). Het probleem van de seksualiteit. Wat is het probleem? *Tijdschrift voor Psychoanalyse en haar toepassingen, 28*, 254–264.
19 Freud, S. (1909). Notes upon a case of obsessional neurosis. In *Freud standard edition* (p. 201). London: Hogarth.
20 De Waal, F. (2007). *De aap en de filosoof.* Antwerpen-Amsterdam: Contact.
21 Kinet, M. (2023). *The spirit of the drive in neuropsychoanalysis.* London/New York: Routledge.
22 Vroon, P. (1989). *De tranen van de krokodil.* Baarn: Ambo.
23 Linden, E. (1986). *Silent partners: The legacy of the ape language experiments.* New York: Times Books.
24 Savage-Rumbaugh, S., & Lewin, R. (1994). *Kanzi: The ape at the brink of the human mind.* New York: Wiley.
25 De Waal, F. (2007). *De aap en de filosoof.* Antwerpen-Amsterdam: Contact.
26 Cluckers, G., & Meurs, P. (2005). Bruggen tussen denk-wijzen. In M. Kinet & R. Vermote (Red.), *Mentalisatie.* Antwerpen/Apeldoorn: Garant.
27 Trevarthen, C. (Ed.) (1990). *Brain circuits and functions of the mind.* Cambridge: Cambridge University Press.
28 Freud, S. (1916–1917). *Colleges inleiding tot de psychoanalyse I.P.1 /2. Sigmund Freud, Nederlandse Editie.* Amsterdam/Meppel: Boom.
29 Freud, S. (1913/2006). *Totem en taboe: Enkele overeenkomsten in het psychische leven van wilden en neurotici* (R. Kooistra, Vert.). Amsterdam: Boom.
30 Rorty, R. (1989). *Contingency, irony, solidarity.* London: Cambridge University Press.
31 Chimpanzee Sequencing and Analysis Consortium. Waterson, R. H., Lander, E. S., & Wilson, R. K. (2005). Initial sequence of the chimpanzee genome and comparison with the human genome. *Nature, 437*(7055), 69–87.
32 Lacan, J. (1949/1966). Le stade du miroir comme formateur de la fonction du Je. In *Ecrits* (pp. 93–100). Paris: Du Seuil.
33 Dawkins, R. (1997). *The selfish gene.* New York: Norton.
34 Mülisch, H. (1990). Oedipus als Freud. In *de Zuilen van Hercules.* Amsterdam: Bezige Bij.
35 https://fcmconference.org/img/CambridgeDeclarationOnConsciousness.pdf

8

The Square of Desire

Oedipus

In classical Freudian theory, the Oedipus complex is not only the core complex of neurosis, but also of our love lives.[1] Our identities and relationships are structured around it. From a psychoanalytic perspective, the way we pass through this 'mountain pass' is of great significance for our gender identity and sexual orientation, as well as for our moral development as civilised beings. The Oedipus complex thus provides an initial, foundational symbolic structure.[2] Depending on time and culture, it takes on different forms and is embodied in various figures with differing functions. In Lacanian terms, the Big Other inscribes itself in the psyche. It lodges itself between skin and flesh and makes of us, in the words of Aristotle, a *zoön politikon*, a political animal.[3] Family must not be reduced to biological kinship, but is a configuration of mutual relations, commands and prohibitions, rights and duties, which vary according to time and culture, especially concerning who may enjoy what, how, and from whom. In more familiar language: the Big Other determines what we may or may not find pleasurable – in the kitchen, the living room, the bedroom, and in public life.[4]

We do not pass through the Oedipus complex unscathed. Inevitably, we emerge from it with bruises and abrasions. Naturally, we contort ourselves in various ways to avoid discomfort, such that, in an unexpected turn, through the so-called pleasure principle, we end up entangled with ourselves. For the child's optimal psychological development, love among the parents is probably more important than the parental love for the child. When the parental couple has an unsatisfying relationship, a skewed triangle can emerge in which one or both parents seek emotional fulfilment through the child. The child is then insufficiently confronted with loving parents as a sexual couple. Instead, the child aligns more closely with one parent and may come to believe that it can or must satisfy that parent's desires. The boundaries between the sexes, between generations, and those surrounding the incest taboo become blurred.

What is missing here is the paternal function (not to be confused with the father as person), which must act as a third term – both prohibiting and protecting. Ideally, this function curbs the boundless love that can pathologically entangle parent and child. What is at stake here are universal desires, and the child must be lovingly

DOI: 10.4324/9781003728764-8

'put in its place' in order to establish a proper triangular structure. When this triangulation functions well, the child is confronted with boundaries and desires that free them from the illusion of their centrality. This has a protective value: it sets the child in its rightful place. Parental love can be so overwhelming that the law or limits are no longer respected, out of fear of losing the child's affection. In such cases, development shifts from *education* to *seduction*, thereby establishing a Kingdom of the Child. Some pessimists see this as one of the ailments of our time.[5]

Square

The Oedipus complex is essential for understanding certain characteristics and problems in love. Love and infatuation depend heavily on the structure or context in which they arise. One is in love as long as the partner remains unreachable or forbidden. But once a couple is together and love becomes a sort of duty, the intensity of feeling often fades. Living together in a 'nation of two,' it all seems idyllic: *I only have eyes for you, baby*. The wish for children is seen as the cherry on top. But once the newborn has descended from heaven, a fatal finale suddenly appears from nowhere. Nothing works smoothly anymore. Desire starts turning square.

But no need to worry, because as soon as one of the partners falls for a third party, desire flares up once again. In all these cases, nothing intrinsic about the partner has changed – only the configuration in which the love relationship is embedded.

This is not visible to the naked eye, but we are no longer dealing with a triangular structure – rather, it has become square. In the Oedipal context, the boy tries to possess that 'something' the father appears to have, which causes the mother to prefer him: money, physical strength, social status, humour, intellect, or simply a larger penis. Mutatis mutandis, the mother, too, seems to possess seductive qualities for the father that the girl lacks: sexual attributes such as hair, lips, gaze, or the classic trio of belly, breasts, and buttocks; but also culinary skills, class, charisma, or caregiving abilities.

These descriptions are, of course, somewhat 'classical' – sex appeal may just as well be based on subtler traits. The father might be a 'bandit' or a rebel without a cause. The mother may exude artistic flair or be a full-blown drama queen. That *something* the other has or is, Lacan calls the phallus, and we are endlessly in search of this presumed key to success.

Some love problems can become highly symptomatic. A certain pattern repeats itself, and the roots must be unearthed if the person involved is ever to be freed from it. An acquaintance, for instance, took devilish pleasure in repeatedly seducing his friends' partners. The thrill of the challenge fed his desire, and competition with other men quickened his pulse. A married woman, meanwhile, moved from lover to lover, each of whom she persuaded to pay for various things. In this way, she sought revenge on her father, who had once placed her on a pedestal, only to abandon her mercilessly after the birth of another child. In both cases, an Oedipal scenario is playing out – without the 'actors' being consciously aware of it.

Mum and Dad

Most people readily acknowledge that their parents exerted a significant influence on their emotional development. Few grasp the full extent of this influence. Crucially, we are not discussing the parents as they are today, but as they appeared to the child's developing eyes. Both the parents and the image we hold of them are dynamic and evolve over time. Broadly speaking, the 'object representations' we carry in our heads grow in shading, dimension, and complexity.

On the anaclitic pole of partner choice, the selection is based on self-preservative drives – such as the need for warmth, nourishment, and care. The partner matches a parental imago and is cherished, respected, and obeyed, if not idealised. There is great love but little desire. According to Freud, only a minority of men succeed in combining tender and erotic feelings.[6] For the vast majority, early erotic impulses (of an oral, anal, or genital nature) were already triggered in relation to the mother or other intimate family members. Initially, the child felt innocent regarding these early sexual feelings. Only *nachträglich* (retroactively) are they experienced as dirty, impure, or bad, once the child has become aware of the sexual (incest) taboo. Just as urine and faeces were only found to be disgusting at a later stage, so erotic feelings acquire their 'dirty' connotation in retrospect.

There are times when a therapist knows precisely how their patients fail in love, and in the evening the therapist fails in precisely the same way. Not because the therapist doesn't know better, but because this knowledge does not exempt them from repetition.

American Lacanian Bruce Fink writes beautifully about (pre-Oedipal) Mum 1 and (Oedipal) Mum 2.[7] At first, there is the innocent child and his Madonna: the pure, virginal mother. Only after the 'fall' appears Mum 2 – the whorish mother, perverse or exploitative. Mum 1 denied the father sexual privilege; Mum 2 is the sinful mother who ultimately betrays or deceives her son.[8] It is difficult to see Mum 1 and Mum 2 as one and the same woman. Hence, a male impasse often noted by Freud: where he loves, he does not desire; where he desires, he does not love.[9] He 'falls' for a sweet girl, courts her in due form, and behaves like a cautious elephant in a China shop. The girl is a successor to the mother, or is transformed into Mum 1, especially when she herself becomes a mother in the literal sense. Meanwhile, he desires a 'bad' woman, meaning that she offers extra-legal benefits and seems willing to cross moral or legal boundaries. It is entirely possible that he fantasises about rescuing this woman from the clutches of alcohol, drugs, or predatory men, in an effort to transform Mum 2 back into Mum 1.

Freud's advice to men: anyone who wishes to love freely and happily must overcome his respect for women and come to terms with his incestuous fantasies.[10] Fink is less certain about women. According to Princess Marie Bonaparte (Freud's analysand, pupil, and later benefactor who helped him emigrate to London), the question remained a mystery to him: *Was will das Weib?* Women, it seems, have less need to devalue their love object in order to enjoy sex freely. Nor do they idealise their partner in quite the same way. Alongside Prince Charming and Mr Right, they may well be attracted to the macho *bad boy* who acts brusquely and does not treat her like a princess.

In contemporary neuropsychoanalytic terms, the Oedipus complex marks the first emergence of intense inner conflicts between ATTACHMENT/GRIEF, CARE, and LUST. These systems are mirrored, encouraged, or, conversely, prohibited to varying degrees. Secure attachment, concern for offspring, and sexual drive are intrinsically at odds with one another, even outside the imperatives of the Big Other. Nevertheless, any choice or compromise is better than none at all, and decisions must be made (often for reasons of psychic energy conservation) before every knot is untangled. These decisions create folds – psychic creases – which may come back to trouble us later in life.[11]

Love Lacks

From a more philosophical-anthropological perspective, all human desire revolves around a lack: a mythical enjoyment that was forfeited when the child was weaned from the breast, subjected to toilet training, and pushed from the mother's lap. In so-called symbolic castration, we are separated from the maternal Thing by language and the Name-of-the-Father. All desire stems from the endless displacement caused by this *manque-à-être* – this lack of being.[12] In English, this is variably translated into a 'want-to-be' or a 'wannabe' – the phallus.

To love is to give what one does not have. Love is a gesture of lack: an offering of something one oneself is missing. You cannot explain it – you do not know what it is – you only know that something is absent. To truly love someone is to tell them, in words, that you are missing something, and that this person is deeply connected to that lack. I quote Colette Soler: Love is the admission of lack.[13] A degree of symmetry is essential here, for to love is also to wish to be loved.[14] As a beloved, we want to be the ultimate one – the love object that finally halts the endless chain of substitution. We want to be the phallus for the other, or the object *petit a* that sparks the other's desire.

Loving desire presupposes not only the recognition of a lack, but also the capacity to elevate one's beloved to the dignity of the Thing. In doing so, the interchangeability of partners comes to an end, and the lovers can finally say to one another: *You are the One.*

Notes

1 Freud, S. (1931). Over de vrouwelijke seksualiteit. K.B.3. *Sigmund Freud Nederlandse Editie* (p. 126). Amsterdam/Meppel: Boom.
2 Green, A. (1992). Oedipe, Freud et nous. In A. Green (Ed.), *La déliaison* (pp. 69–147). Paris: Hachette.
3 Ackrill, J. L. (1994). *Aristoteles*. Groningen: Historische Uitgeverij.
4 Kinet, M. (2019). Enkele oedipale variaties. Van Darwin tot Lacan. In M. Kinet & W. Heuves (Red.), *Driehoeksverhoudingen Actuele oedipale variaties* (pp. 51–70). Antwerpen/'s Hertogenbosch: Gompel&Svacina.

5 Marcelli D. (2003). *L'enfant, chef de la famille*. Paris: Albin Michel.
6 Freud, S. (1912). On the universal tendency to debasement in the sphere of love. In *Freud standard edition* (Vol. 2, p. 180). London. Hogarth Press.
7 Fink, B. (2015). *Lacan on love: An exploration of Lacan's Seminar VIII, Transference*. New York: Polity.
8 Freud, S. (1910). A special type of object choice made by men. In *Freud standard edition* (Vol. 2, pp. 168–170). London. Hogarth Press.
9 Freud, S. (1912). On the universal tendency to debasement in the sphere of love. In *Freud standard edition* (Vol. 2, p. 183). London. Hogarth Press.
10 Freud, S. (1912). On the universal tendency to debasement in the sphere of love. In *Freud standard edition* (Vol. 2, p. 186). London. Hogarth Press.
11 Solms M. (2021). A revision of Freud's theory of the biological origin of the oedipus complex. *Psychoanalytic Quaterly*, *90*(4), 555–581.
12 Lacan, J. (1958/1966). La direction de la cure et les principes de son pouvoir. In *Ecrits* (p. 623). Paris: Seuil.
13 Soler, C. (2003). *Ce que Lacan disait des femmes* (p. 243). Paris: Champ Lacanien.
14 Lacan, J. (1966). La science et la vérité. In *Ecrits* (p. 853). Paris: Seuil.

9

Biologised Love

Science and Literature

Trust, faith, hope, and love are evidently vital. They play a decisive role not only in the survival of the individual but also in that of the species. And yet science has little time for such sentiments. Since Karl Popper, science has been bound to the ideals of measurability and falsifiability. What lies beyond that boundary belongs to the realm of literature.[1] History, sociology, and anything related to the psyche are seen as the playground of artists and philosophers, while scientists amuse themselves with elementary particles or black holes. The gulf between the life we live with heart and soul, and the realm of measurable, experimentally manipulable events, thus becomes as vast – metaphorically speaking – as the one between string and superstring.

Psychiatry and Psychoanalysis

Medicine, as is well known, is an applied natural science. It is characterised by a clinic of the gaze. For medicine, only what can be seen is real: in blood, urine, or other bodily fluids, through various types of 'imaging', or via an eye at the end of a snake-like instrument that can penetrate the deepest cavities of the body. When nothing can be seen, medicine speaks of non-objectifiable complaints. These are, notably, the daily bread of every GP's practice. They are attributed either to the nerves or labelled with the (evasive) diagnosis of 'idiopathic.' A scholarly word to take out into society, which merely means: inexplicable.

Psychiatry, as a subspecialty of medicine, straddles both the natural and the human sciences. Some speak of this awkward position as a split, or more elegantly, a *grand écart.* Within the psychoanalytic world, views differ on the status of psychoanalysis. The Anglophone tradition grants it a role similar to that of psychiatry, while the Latin school emphasises its irreducibly cultural nature, repeatedly insisting on the anthropological difference. Yet, for every psychoanalyst, it is essentially a science of the particular and/or of the subjective/subject.

It is characterised, first and foremost, by a clinic of the ear. The unconscious exists only for those who 'listen' to it. Some formations of the unconscious

DOI: 10.4324/9781003728764-9

include the (day)dream, the slip of the tongue, the impulsive act, and the symptom. This symptom is not to be understood, as in medicine, as a mere sign of disease, but as a signifier. It is a narrative element whose meaning emerges only within its synchronic and diachronic contexts. More precisely, the (psychoanalytic) symptom is an involuntary phenomenon that recurs, from which the subject suffers but which, covertly, also provides some gain or enjoyment, and which poses a question (of translation) addressed to the Other. Not only feelings of inferiority or agoraphobia, but also a specific passion or partner choice may function as symptoms. What all these formations share is that they are openings through which something of the fissure within our being becomes visible. They show that we are not masters of our own house, and that something within us can take over control despite our best intentions or rational awareness.

Medicine has no desire to engage with any of this. According to Michel Foucault, it derives its power precisely from the privileging of a discourse based on objectifiable, measurable observations (the so-called *mathesis*) over other discourses, such as those grounded in introspection.[2] As one of its youngest offspring, psychiatry has, in recent decades, sought to be as medical as possible in order to be granted a seat at the table with the 'grown-ups.' Today, many psychiatrists are virtually brain scientists – technicians who predominantly remove symptoms by biological means. Yet, by definition, symptoms are surface phenomena: the proverbial tip of the iceberg that conceals deeper processes from view.

Neuroscience

This evolution is closely linked to the rapid growth of neuroscience. As early as 450 BCE, Hippocrates located the realm of emotion in the brain. In the nineteenth century, Wilhelm Griesinger held that all mental disorders were brain disorders – a biologically reductionist view that has regained ground in recent decades.[3] The reasons are twofold. Psychotropic drugs were only introduced after the Second World War. These had spectacular effects on major psychiatric disorders, which had previously been almost entirely untreatable. The disordered neurotransmitter activity discovered since then has been held responsible for most mental illnesses. Gross simplifications are the rule here. To use an analogy: just because aspirin works for fever and headache does not mean that these are caused – let alone solely caused – by a lack of aspirin. Did the Stone Age come to an end because we ran out of stones?

Above all, the popularity of so-called biological psychiatry is due to spectacular technological research and its resulting applications. This includes the molecular biology of neural tissue, memory research, computer models, cyber applications, and artificial intelligence. Current brain imaging (SPECT scan, fMRI) allows us to visualise not only the brain's anatomical structure, but also its functioning – even during the most intimate and subjective mental processes. Every doubting Thomas can now witness the mind with his own eyes...

At the macroscopic level, we observe two hemispheres that, like a walnut, rest upon the underlying brainstem. Each hemisphere consists of four lobes, each with its own functional profile. In simplified terms and moving from back to front: the occipital lobe governs vision, the parietal lobe is responsible for three-dimensional spatial orientation, the temporal lobe handles hearing and emotional perception, while the frontal lobe oversees morality, wisdom, and ambition – those 'higher' functions involving values and ideals.

Microscopically, the brain appears to be an exceptional organ that continuously reshapes itself in response to its environment. A child's brain is still in full development after birth, and up until (young) adulthood, we can observe a progressive furrowing of the forehead and the darkening – becoming 'wiser' – of the neocortex behind it.

In general, and particularly with respect to brain development, genetic predisposition manifests only through interaction with environmental factors. This neuroplasticity occurs through cross-wiring and continuous neuronal interconnectivity. Hardware and software interact in a constant, inseparable manner. Memory is divided into implicit and explicit forms, which emerge successively in early life, with the former offering no stricto sensu capacity for recollection. Many of our motor, sensory, cognitive, and emotional processes run simultaneously through higher (neo-)cortical and lower limbic or subcortical systems, often proceeding phenomenologically unconsciously. These are just a few examples from the extensive findings of contemporary neuroscience.

Neuropsychoanalysis

In the year 2000 – the symbolic Year Zero of this third millennium – Mark Solms founded the *International Neuropsychoanalysis Society*.[4] Its adherents hope that this new interdisciplinary science might provide a theory of everything for the mind, just as string theory aspires to do for physics. Admittedly, the latter requires ten hypothetical dimensions to make this work…

In such a framework, neuropsychoanalysis could offer an integration of brain science with sustained attention to subjective experience. It would thus avoid the pitfalls of simplistic, mechanistic reductions and the murky mythologising of the drive-based psyche. Its aim is a metapsychology grounded in the bodily substrate. In this respect, neuropsychoanalysis distinguishes itself from more evolutionarily biological or psychological approaches, which are often dismissed as too speculative. These tend to exhibit a striking lack of experimentation and observation, as well as minimal engagement with or exploration of inner life.

Although self-assured and full of promise, neuropsychoanalysis is (still?) highly contested. In a dialogue between Jacques-Alain Miller and Horacio Etchegoyen – two leading figures of mutually exclusive psychoanalytic schools – the former put it somewhat polemically: 'And what if our mind had its correlate in the mind of God?'[5] He considers such neuro-correlations entirely devoid of clinical relevance. Others (including the Belgian Lacanian Ariane Bazan), use abundant neuroscientific findings to support Lacan's dictum regarding the linguistic structure of the unconscious – and of the brain.[6] Neuroscience, too, shows that there is a knowledge within us that we do not (or cannot or will not) know. This is at times due to the peculiarities of certain memory circuits (cannot?), and at others to the inhibitory (want not?) effects of the neocortex and/or left hemisphere.

Of Love

In the domain of love research, neuropsychology still faces significant limitations. It emphasises the study of higher cortical functions at the expense of lower (epi-) limbic ones. These cortical areas are, after all, more accessible – but that does not necessarily mean they are more important. According to Solms, there is, in any case, a knowledge gap regarding the brain's instinctual domain compared to the regions where the ego is believed to reside.[7]

And yet, our happiness depends to a great extent on our capacity to discover a hidden world – one that turns, invisibly, improbably, and irrepressibly, around love. It is love that fosters lasting relationships marked by such features as attachment, commitment, intimacy, passion, grief upon separation, jealousy, and so forth – traits that can also, to a certain degree, be recognised in some higher mammals. In the dual phase of attraction and attachment, an emotional bond can develop with someone whose absence is felt and with whom sensory stimuli are exchanged in cycles of desire, satisfaction, satiety, aversion, and renewed desire. Hunger is the best sauce. 'Love' is stirred by the cycle of frustration and gratification. Several neurobiologists point to a connection with the economy of desire – so-called 'reward' systems – as well as with the pathways of feeding and addiction in the brain. Selfless motherly love is a universal myth or archetype, and people fight fiercely to obtain or preserve it.

Brain imaging also shows that romantic and parental love are both distinct and overlapping.[8] The latter is located in areas where the transmission and metabolism of oxytocin and vasopressin predominate. This is also accompanied by a deactivation of areas responsible for social judgment and mentalisation, casting the phenomenon of love's blindness in a new, neural light.[9]

Falling in love increases stress and cortisol levels in our bodies. Yet, happiness, pleasure, touch, social contact, and emotional support – all part of love – provide, conversely, a neurobiologically demonstrable sense of safety and a reduction in stress. Biologised love appears to be a complex phenomenon, resting on the foundation of attachment and the trust it implies, while simultaneously being governed by motivational 'reward' systems – both appetitive (pleasure-seeking) and aversive (pain-avoiding).[10]

Love Drive?

But is there, biologically speaking, such a thing as a 'love drive'? Based on neuroscientific and evolutionary evidence, Helen Fisher argues for a specific drive underlying romantic love.[11] According to her, attraction and partner selection stem from an autonomous emotional system separate from both sexuality and attachment. It is this system that produces the characteristic focus on one specific partner, the desire to follow, affectionate gestures, jealousy (which evolutionary biologists term 'mate guarding'), and the powerful motivation to fight for the preferred partner.

If we understand the drive as a more rudimentary category than the instinct – which is bound to specific emotional and behavioural repertoires – neuropsychoanalyst Yoram Yovell remains unconvinced. For him, the LUST and ATTACHMENT (or PANIC-GRIEF) systems, when sufficiently fuelled by the more general SEEKING system, are entirely sufficient to explain romantic love. In their entanglement, these components, for him, suffice.[12]

Biologised

The reader will undoubtedly have recognised much that feels 'natural' in the preceding lines. It all sounds reasonable and transparent. And yet, this straightforward logic does not entirely correspond to the reality encountered in the psychoanalyst's consulting room. It is the difference between a dream and (in this case) clinical reality. As Freud discovered, the dream protects sleep.[13] Through distortion and concealment, it does everything in its power to prevent the sleeper from waking. Psychoanalysis aspires to the exact opposite. Its 'dream' is that of radical awakening. And so it dares to ask the most troubling questions.

Why does someone remain, for years, the hostage of an impossible love? Why does another yearn for the unattainable? Why can love drive people to joint suicide – or to a *folie à deux*? Why do lovers write letters and poems to each other rather than consummate their desire? What is it, really, that we see in the beloved – against all better judgment? What if absence is love's only true gift? Is love not above all a hymn to an erected object which, once attained, deflates and dissolves?

As a deceptive mirroring, love is essentially a form of deception, says Jacques Lacan.[14] There is no need to biologise love – for it is love that biologises us. Love rarely marches in straight lines. We are bound to the Other by something – by a Thing. But this Thing binds us only if we keep it at a distance. To seek the Thing in the other is already to undo the bond. The enjoyment of love is intrinsically destructive. Desire and longing are directed towards it, but we cannot truly be present with it. Our orgasm is all the more intense the more we lose ourselves in it. When we truly listen to what unfolds in love stories, we find little rationality. On the contrary, they are overflowing with sense, nonsense, and madness.

Notes

1 Popper, K. R. (1963). *Conjectures and refutations*. London: Routledge.
2 Foucault, M. (1961). *Histoire de la folie à l'âge classique*. Paris: Gallimard.
3 Hoff, P., & Hippius, H. (2001). Wilhelm Griesinger (1817–1868) – sein Psychiatrieverständnis aus historischer und aktueller Perspektive. *Der Nervenarzt, 72*, 885–892.
4 Kinet. (2024). *The spirit of the drive in neuropsychoanalysis*. London/New York: Routledge.

5 Etchegoyen, R. H. et Miller, J. A. (1996). *Silence Brisé. Entretien sur le mouvement psychanalytique*. Paris: Agalma Diffusion Seuil.
6 Bazan, A. (2011). Phantoms in the voice. A neuropsychoanalytic hypothesis on the structure of the unconscious. *Neuropsychoanalysis*, *13*(2), 161–176.
7 Kinet. (2024). *The spirit of the drive in neuropsychoanalysis*. London/New York: Routledge.
8 Fisher, H. E., Aron, A., & Brown, L. L. (2005). Romantic love: An fMRI study of a neural mechanism for mate choice. *Journal of Comparative Neurology*, *493*(1), 58–62.
9 Bartels, A., & Zeki, S. (2000). The neural basis of romantic love. *NeuroReport*, *11*(17), 3829–3834.
10 Zeki, S. (2007). The neurobiology of love. *FEBS Letters*, *581*(14), 2575–2579.
11 Fisher, H. (2004). *Why we love*. New York: Holt.
12 Yovell, Y. (2008). Is there a drive to love? *Neuropsychoanalysis*, *10*(2), 140.
13 Freud, S. (1900). *De droomduiding. P.D.2/3. Sigmund Freud Nederlandse Editie* (pp. 1–713). Amsterdam/Meppel: Boom.
14 Lacan, J. (1975). *Le Séminaire Livre XX. Encore*. Texte établi par J. A. Miller. Paris: Du Seuil.

Panoramic Intermezzo I

Love first appears not as a story but as a movement.
Not as a possession but as a verb.
Not as a relationship but as a coming-into-being.

In this first movement of the book, we see how love detaches itself from the biological and immediately inscribes itself in language, gaze, body and desire. The child who longs to be loved, the lover who succumbs, the animal that attaches, the human being who dreams, the species that organises itself — these are not separate figures but variations of a single grammar: a subject who does not possess itself and who seeks in the other something that can never be fully given.

What takes shape here is not a psychology but a structure.

Love reveals itself not as a sentiment but as a necessary fiction through which the human animal learns to live with lack.
It forms itself between instinct and meaning, between nature and culture, between neurobiology and symbolism.

The desire that emerges is never purely biological, never purely cultural: it is always already split, always already mediated, always already in relation to something that is missing.

Thus, in this first arc, the fundamental tone is set: love is not an answer to life, but the way in which life poses its questions.

DOI: 10.4324/9781003728764-10

10

Love between Neuro and Meta

Satisfaction

As recently as 2019, the twentieth congress of the *International Neuropsychoanalysis Society* took place in Brussels under the title 'Satisfaction at Last: Neuropsychoanalysis on Sex, Drive, and Enjoyment.' Around the same time, I also published on the spirit of the drive within neuropsychoanalysis, integrating and critically discussing the work of its founding father, Mark Solms and of my compatriot Ariane Bazan, with their respective Freudian and Lacanian foundations.[1] Can a neuroscientific perspective on love and sexuality still be overlooked today? The question answers itself.

If we begin, for example, by examining the sexual response cycle developed by Masters and Johnson, we observe an initial increase in energy and enthusiasm during which other stimuli are ignored, directing attention exclusively to the desired object. In the second, plateau phase, arousal and desire increase further. The third, orgasmic phase brings intense pleasure and a full-body release, particularly centred in the genitals. Finally, there is a fourth, so-called refractory phase, in which energy drops, relaxation sets in, and feelings of closeness and affection towards the partner become paramount. The first two and the last two phases correspond, respectively, to Jaak Panksepp's SEEKING/WANTING[2] and Kent Berridge's LIKING systems.[3] Each phase provides a different form of enjoyment: anticipatory and consummatory, jouissance and plaisir.

The first kind of pleasure is linked to appetite ('appetitive'), the second to consumption ('consummatory'). Each phase involves distinct neuroanatomical and neurochemical systems: in chronological order, dopamine, vasopressin, endogenous opioids, and finally the so-called 'cuddle hormone' oxytocin.[4] During orgasm, there is an overlap between WANTING and LIKING, accompanied by corresponding peaks in their respective neurochemistry. There are, moreover, many different forms of pleasure, each associated with its respective affective systems.[5]

Lacan, by contrast, introduced the dialectic among *besoin* (need), *demande* (demand), and *désir* (desire).[6] A need can only be expressed in the form of a demand, which, beyond merely seeking the satisfaction of the need, also includes a plea for love. One can nourish an infant through a feeding tube or an intravenous drip.

DOI: 10.4324/9781003728764-11

This may satisfy the physical need for food and hydration, but it does not fulfil the demand, and certainly not the desire. Desire is quintessentially human. It superimposes itself upon and also transcends the demand. The demand is gradually articulated in the code or language of the big Other – namely, the mother tongue. Yet, desire gravitates around an enigmatic signifier that crystallises out of the imaginary: the phallus, as that which one can never (fully) possess or become in order to completely satisfy the desire of the Other.

Desire emerges in the gap between need and demand. Or rather, it appears at the threshold where the demand is subtracted from the need. In need, we appeal to or direct a demand towards the big Other. The Other's response inevitably falls short of or overshoots what was requested, thereby causing a 'surplus' that is constitutive of desire.

We may articulate our needs as precisely and thoroughly as we like, but our demand must pass through the narrow bottleneck of language and in doing so, it gives rise to that most distinctively human phenomenon: desire. Indeed, it is all 'merely psychic.'

Sex Essentials

In line with this, I expand on what Ariane Bazan considers essential to sexuality.[7] Air, food, water, or faeces are examples of pre-genital objects that bring about gratification through pleasure, jouissance, and affect. A deficit within the internal body (a need) can be remedied, and an adequate action is possible. In the case of erogenous zones, there is no homeostatic criterion originating within the body. It is (merely) the motor action that brings pleasure, and a fully adequate action is impossible. For Bazan, the motor action (the signifier being, in the first instance, an articulated motor pattern) may lead to relief in three ways: active, passive, and reflexive (wherein the subject takes itself as the object – Freud's auto-eroticism). She also emphasises the importance of the big Other, the symbolic order that permeates all objects.[8] In this view, the sexual is disconnected from any homeostatic anchor point, and its architecture is determined by a symbolic order that governs the regulation of tension.

Although it is highly recommended, it falls outside the scope of this chapter to follow Bazan's argument in full. Still, I will briefly summarise how she distinguishes the non-sexual from the sexual. In the non-sexual, the source of the drive lies in the internal vegetative systems of the (smooth-muscle) inner body. Here, satisfaction takes the form of a restoration of homeostasis – concerning blood sugar, temperature, oxygen levels, and so forth. The object of the non-sexual drive is universal and cannot be represented. It must deliver real satisfaction. The initiation of the nonsexual drive arises from tension in biological membranes. The action involved consists of either providing or removing a material element, thereby enabling an adequate response and fulfilling the need.

Sexuality, by contrast, is situated in the (striated-muscle) surface body (which in vertebrates evolved on top of the inner body) and within the erogenous zones (defined by Bazan as particularly where the inner and surface body intersect). In sexuality, pleasure arises solely from the motor discharge of tension or arousal. Erogenous or sexual objects are singular and emerge through the contingent history of the subject. They are representable and, in Lacanian terms, belong not to the Real but to the symbolic-imaginary. Sexual initiation, then, derives on the one hand from tactile stimulation of the genitalia and erogenous zones. Interestingly, men reportedly have the same erogenous zones as women, but in women these zones are more sensitive[9] – perhaps a neuropsychoanalytic correlate of the feminine jouissance (‘*supplémentaire*’) that is not governed by the (phallic) pleasure principle.

Another source of sexual arousal lies in representations, originating from one's own mental activity and/or from that of the big Other. In sexuality, an adequate action is impossible, because symbolic and logical (as opposed to material) principles are at work: it is the symbolic-imaginary that exerts its influence. Here, pleasure is a more appropriate term than satisfaction. It is not only The Rolling Stones who ‘can't get no satisfaction.’

Exciting

Jouissance is arousal. It correlates with the SEEKING system and is accompanied by a dopamine spike in the nucleus accumbens, our pleasure centre. Jouissance may be experienced as pleasurable or painful. Bazan broadly argues that a release of dopamine signals that the body has been surprised – something has happened in or to it. Pleasure, on the other hand, entails the release of internal opioids and corresponds with a pleasurable affect: LIKING. According to Bazan, pleasure and jouissance may combine in varying mixtures. One can be satisfied without jouissance and experience jouissance without pleasurable affect.

But this dopamine release also has further effects on the body. The dopamine spike reinforces the behaviours that the organism engaged in at the time of the surprise or event. This phenomenon, called ‘incentive salience,’ ensures that the motor patterns associated with the surprise or event are recorded in the brain.[10] The operative motor schemas undergo molecular and cellular changes, enabling them to be activated more quickly, easily, and forcefully whenever a future cue recalls the event.

The movements that historically led the organism to satisfaction (of the inner body) or pleasure (in the surface body) are inscribed in such a way that the organism is driven to repeat them. When something reminds the subject of the original event, central activation and peripheral tension build up. The release of this activation and the discharge of this tension become pleasurable in themselves, regardless of whether the outcome of the action is satisfactory or not. The essence of sex thus stems from particular representations and the direct stimulation of erogenous zones. It is tied to the enjoyment of the act itself and gives rise to the contingent ‘objects’ unique to the narrative of the singular subject.

Rocket Science

The subject may relate to this object actively or passively, but through the organising dynamic of language (that is, in a reflexive mode) it can also become the object itself. From this neuro-logical line of thought, we now ascend to a more philosophical meta-logic. This stratosphere will inevitably reduce oxygen levels; therefore, the reader is advised to take a deep breath. Light-headedness cannot be excluded, though it may be alleviated.

What, for example, does the Slovenian philosopher and psychoanalyst Alenka Zupančič discuss in her book *What is Sex?*[11] She criticises the way we speak about sex as though we know what we are talking about. Sex, she argues, is systematically reduced to a self-evident phenomenon marked by positive and observable features – features that are deemed problematic only because they are caught between prohibitive conservatism on one side and progressive liberalisation on the other. Yet, according to Zupančič, this shifting social context conceals a dialectic that is intrinsic to sexuality itself. Sex is not, for her, a pre-discursive entity that ought to be regulated in this or that way. It is precisely for this reason that we are so obsessed with it – even when we claim to want to rid ourselves of it. External taboos or restrictions surrounding sexuality tend, in her view, to obscure its (not positive but) negative core.

In Zupančič's account, the unconscious is itself a sexualised mode of thinking. Freud did not merely uncover the importance of sexuality ('sex is not everything, but it is *in* everything'); he revealed its inherent problem. The sexual unconscious is not so much a repository of dirty secrets as it is simply the way the mind operates. For this reason, sex is a curious entity. It is marked by negativity. It cannot be known. Sex is an ultimate enigma, a shadow realm that nonetheless demands to be endlessly spoken about. Sex is not something that exists beforehand and is then put into words. On the contrary, it emerges from the paradoxical and dual movement of discourse itself. Through its gestures of concealment and revelation, this discourse testifies to an inherent contradiction. As its signifiers become more rarefied, this effect may be somewhat mitigated.

Subcutaneous

For Lacan, the unconscious does not lie in the depths as a realm of repressed feelings or desires. It comes from outside, from the big Other, from language, and from social structures that exist beyond us, embedding themselves between skin and flesh (*'entre cuir et chair'*).[12] The unconscious is the discourse of the big Other; it is invasive, arriving from elsewhere. A dimension of repression is already built into this discourse itself. Language is structured as repression, because the word is a presence made of an absence (*'une présence faite d'absence'*).[13] It wrestles with its own impossibility.

Sex, for Zupančič, is tied up with this very structure. The order of signifiers arises with (or from) a lack of signifier that is, as it were, built into the system: the *hiatus sexualis*.[14] The chain of signifiers is incomplete. The symbolic order begins not with 1, but – figuratively speaking – with -1. In Lacanian theory, the phallus functions first and foremost as the signifier of lack and of (symbolic) castration. It represents a structural minus.

That Lacan chooses the phallic signifier is therefore not because men happen to possess a phallus. He by no means intends to idealise a merely coincidental male characteristic. It would be a mistake to replace the phallus with a supposedly more neutral term – or worse still, with a biologically female equivalent like the uterus. Such a substitution would reflect a misguided (and tendentious) reading of phallocentrism. Lacan selects the phallus as the fundamental signifier precisely because half the world's population manifestly does *not* possess this organ. It is this non-immediacy – this *cut* from the organic – that makes the phallus the signifier *par excellence* of a presence made of an absence. The phallus is a heterogeneous element with respect to the order of signifiers, and yet it determines its very grammar.

Minus One

It is precisely at the site of this minus or lack that a surplus of enjoyment (*jouissance)* emerges, which contaminates or disrupts the purity of the signifying chain by 'charging' it with enjoyment. This locus (which at once concerns a surplus of enjoyment and a deficit of signification) embodies a gap that forms the backbone of the drive, and that also drives sexuality.

It is therefore not the case that sex belongs to the body while the signifier belongs to the symbolic order. They both arise from the same source. Sexuality is rooted in the contradiction within the symbolic order itself: in the missing signifier and the excess of enjoyment associated with it. There is an original -1 that gives rise to enjoyment.

We may try to regulate sexual drives and desires – whether through prescriptive norms or prohibitive restrictions – there is always a transgression of this 'hiatus.' We may choose to have more or less sex, but we can never escape the rift at the heart of the sexual domain. The infamous discontent in civilisation is not about the regulation or limitation of drives, but about the curse of language. It is embedded in its inescapable failure – its fatal insufficiency. In Lacan's version of Genesis, the fourth verse is not *fiat lux* but *fiat trou!* Not: let there be light, but: let there be a gap. In a typically provocative pun, cultural philosopher and Lacan scholar Marc De Kesel (alluding to Belgium's most famous criminal) once coined the phrase *Du Trou: X!*[15] – a helpful mnemonic, to be sure.

Notes

1 Kinet, M. (2023). *The spirit of the drive in neuropsychoanalysis*. London/New York: Routledge.

2 Panksepp, J. (1998). *Affective neuro-science: The foundations of human and animal emotions*. New York: Oxford University Press.

3 Berridge, K. C. (1996). Food reward: Brain substrates of wanting and liking. *Neuroscience & Biobehavioral Review, 20*, 1–25.
4 Mosri, F. D. (2019). Report on the 20th congress of the international neuropsychoanalysis society, Brussels, Belgium, 2019: 'Satisfaction at last: Neuropsychoanalysis on sex, drive, and enjoyment'. *Neuropsychoanalysis, 21*(2), 139–159.
5 Lacan, J. (1956–1957/1994). *Le Séminaire Livre IV. La relation d'objet*. Texte établi par Jacques-Alain Miller. Paris: Seuil.
6 Mosri, F. D. (2019). Report on the 20th congress of the international neuropsychoanalysis society, Brussels, Belgium, 2019: 'Satisfaction at last: Neuropsychoanalysis on sex, drive, and enjoyment'. *Neuropsychoanalysis, 21*(2), 140.
7 Bazan, A. (2015). Het wezenlijke van seks. Een metapsychologische denkoefening op het snijvlak tussen neurowetenschap en psychoanalyse. In M. Kinet & K. Baeten (Red.), *Psychoanalyse en/als seksuologie?* (pp. 37–59). Antwerpen/Apeldoorn: Garant.
8 Mosri, F. D. (2019). Report on the 20th congress of the international neuropsychoanalysis society, Brussels, Belgium, 2019: 'Satisfaction at last: Neuropsychoanalysis on sex, drive, and enjoyment'. *Neuropsychoanalysis, 21*(2), 141–143.
9 Mosri, F. D. (2019). Report on the 20th congress of the international neuropsychoanalysis society, Brussels, Belgium, 2019: 'Satisfaction at last: Neuropsychoanalysis on sex, drive, and enjoyment'. *Neuropsychoanalysis, 21*(2), 145. Turnbull, O., Lovett, V., Chaldecott, J., & Lucas, M. (2013). Reports of intimate touch: Erogenous zones and somatosensory cortical organization. *Cortex, 53*, 146–154.
10 Robinson, T. E., & Berridge, K. C. (1993). The neural basis of drug craving: An incentive-sensitization theory of addiction. *Brain Research Reviews, 18*, 247–291.
11 Zupančič, A. (2017). *What is sex?* Cambridge: MIT Press.
12 Lacan, J. (1959–1960/1986). *Le Séminaire. Livre VII. L'éthique de la psychanalyse.* Texte établi par J. A. Miller. Paris: Seuil.
13 Lacan, J. (1953/1966). Fonction et champ de la parole et du langage en psychanalyse. In *Ecrits* (p. 276). Paris: Seuil.
14 Le Gaufey, G. (2013). *Hiatus sexualis. De non-rapport sexuel selon Lacan.* Paris: Epel. en Kinet, M. (2014). Op het scherp van de gulden snede. *Tijdschrift voor Psychoanalyse, 3*, 219–220.
15 De Kesel, M. (1996) *Du Trou: 'X'. Over naastenliefde en psychoanalyse* (Zoomlezing, Sociale Hogeschool Gent d.d. 27/11/1996).

The Ideal of Love

Idealisation

From a psychoanalytic perspective, love is not an ideal, and ideal love does not truly exist. And yet, the state of being in love is a universal human condition in which idealisation takes centre stage. When we fall in love, we relinquish our own subjectivity in favour of a love object that we elevate to the status of sexual ideal. The beloved becomes a *diva,* and the lover longs to be a god in the depths of her thoughts. Idealisation lies at the heart of romantic love, but equally underpins the love between parents and children. If things go somewhat normally, the baby is, for a while, the most beautiful and beloved child in the world; and who were our parents if not almighty gods in the heavens?

Hölderlins famous statement is universal: '*Einmal lebt' ich wie Götter und mehr bedarf's nicht.*'[1] Thanks to such moments of glory, we can feel divine even in the deepest recesses of our minds, even in the most extreme circumstances. Wilfred Bion calls this narcissism essential.[2] It shields us from the most inhuman forms of pain and deprivation.

An excessive and/or persistent concern with attaining ideal love may itself be a sign of psychopathology. It is, for example, characteristic of narcissistic personality disorder. In this case, it represents the feminine variant of an excessive preoccupation with power, success, wealth, or genius – traits more often associated with male narcissism. As Freud paraphrased, fame and honour – at least in the imagination – also lead to the love of women.

The ideal of love assumes the existence of a perfect soulmate – someone who fits like a lid on a pot. The fantasy is that, with this one, everything will work effortlessly, and the loaf will finally be fully baked. And they lived happily ever after. Ingredients of this (day)dream include sweetness and light, white bread, milk, and honey. Love becomes a sugary treat expected to ignite a permanent chain reaction – a core fusion culminating in a meltdown of everlasting bliss.

In Steven Soderbergh's sci-fi film *Solaris,*[3] we see what such indestructible love can actually bring about. Under the influence of the mysterious, animistic super-planet of the same name, George Clooney's character Chris Kelvin finds his life transformed into a nightmare. Love takes on a diabolical quality. It mutates into a

DOI: 10.4324/9781003728764-12

haunting, encircling Medusa from the past – a killer queen who holds him locked within her loving jaws. This nightmare is the dream realised: as in any utopia, once achieved, it inevitably reveals its dystopian underside. According to Bertrand Russell, Thomas More's *Utopia* is both boring and totalitarian. More broadly, he argues, this applies to all utopias, since differences are, for him, essential to happiness.[4]

It is, therefore, just as well that laws and practical obstacles stand between dream and deed. Still, we can understand the melancholy that visits us in the evening, as we prepare to sleep. What protects us from dreams that come true also allows us to keep on desiring. Lack is thus constitutive of desire, and only the law makes this desire possible.

Adolescence

For animals, love is simple. Who has ever heard of an identity crisis in a bull-calf becoming a bull? When an animal is confronted with the opposite sex, it knows what to do. It has an instinct, complete and intact. This instinctive knowledge is inscribed in the Real of genes and chromosomes. The animal knows how it works. It has no questions. It has, of course, no words. It is not required to respond. This purely instinctive knowing is denatured in humans. What is typically human is that immediacy is broken by the Imaginary and the Symbolic. And so, *we do* undergo an adolescent crisis. Its starting gun is the onset of physiological puberty, with its boogie-woogie of hormones. The drive assails us from within; the body undergoes a Kafkaesque transformation. We become truly capable of incest and parricide. That is why we begin going out and separate ourselves from our parents. It may be uncertain whether we are children of Adam and Eve, but at this stage, we are undoubtedly descendants of Narcissus and Oedipus.

Adolescence is, on the one hand, the age of everything still being possible, but on the other, it is precisely the encounter with the impossibility of the Thing, of the drive, of the body. There are many ways to respond to this impossibility: we may choose convention, non-conformity, or invention. But there is no such thing as *The Answer*. There exists no pre-established or predetermined knowledge about the relationship between man and woman, nor about what it means to be a son, daughter, father, or mother. Essentially, the adolescent faces ethical choices.

Adolescence is thus a quest for an answer. Its intellectual dimension may manifest through political or philosophical engagement. Socially, it involves the search for new identifications – whether with idols or among peers. Ultimately, it is an intrapsychic search, a working-through of childhood fantasies. This search is enacted through experience: the adolescent wants to learn by doing. They want (not to obey) but to feel. Their motto is *J'agis donc je suis*: I *act*, therefore I am.

Yet, the 'right' answer is always impossible. It is as elusive as the poet's endless dowsing for the perfect word. This is the eternally failed encounter encapsulated in Lacan's most famous formula: *Il n'y a pas de rapport sexuel* (there is no such thing as a sexual relationship).[5] In one of his characteristic neologisms, Lacan explains that sexuality is neither hetero- nor homosexual, but *hommosexual*.[6] As long as the pursuit of pleasure and enjoyment within interpersonal relations remains central, it is (regardless of gender) in tension with love. After all, everyone harbours particular erotic preferences and fantasies that deviate from the straightforward path of genital sexuality. As Alain de Botton aptly notes, affection rarely survives the transition to the bedroom.[7] Where there is love, there is often neither drive nor desire; where there is bodily desire, there is frequently no love.

In classical psychoanalytic terms, love seeks to fulfil unmet or forbidden childhood wishes. To love and to want to be loved become indistinguishable, and this reciprocity – also seen in friendship – sets love apart from drive, which is one-sided: all excitement and sheer activity. Love, by contrast, is a metaphor. It is misleading and purely imaginary. It creates the illusion of fusion, masking the absence of a sexual relationship. It is based on a dreamed unity with the love object and, by definition, extinguishes desire. Desire, after all, is not aimed at an object, but at a lack. It slips and shifts, always directed elsewhere. It is a metonymy. To quote Marcel Proust: *'Le désir fleurit, la possession flétrit toutes choses.'*[8]

Drive, Duo, Duel

Unlike instinct, which is innate and fixed, drive is variable. Excitement and drive develop this way or that, depending on one's life history. What arouses one person may repel another. Excitement, in any case, centres on certain body parts that unconsciously symbolise the experience of fusion. In erotic desire, sexual arousal also becomes tied to the forbidden and/or impossible incestuous love object. The lover seeks in the other a pleasure that revolves around protrusions and openings, around penetration and invasion. There is a yearning for closeness, for transgressing boundaries, for becoming one.

The erotic satisfaction that arises from rhythmic stimulation symbolises fusion. A psychological and emotional bisexuality emerges, in which the lover also identifies with the other. Two complementary experiences of fusion arise: one finds pleasure in the other's desire and in their response to one's own longing. There is an intersubjective transcendence. The symbolic or fetishist shifting of penetrating and penetrable openings leads to zonal confusion and total body erogeneity.

All of this is accompanied by feelings of transgression on several levels. First, there is the breaking of taboos derived from the Oedipal structure. Every lover, after all, erects an *Arc de Triomphe* over their Oedipal rival. After the initial surge of desire that comes with every new conquest, these incest taboos eventually begin to inhibit flamboyance. Hence, the joke about a special edition of Viagra for married couples: *Viagra Forte.*

Second, there is the transgression vis-à-vis the love object itself, in a boundless game of attraction and repulsion, penetration and surrender. But the most significant transgression is that of the self, which merges with the other, opening not just its story, but exceeding its limits.

According to renowned psychoanalyst Otto Kernberg, sexual arousal in so-called "mature sexual love" is transformed into erotic desire.[9] There is tenderness towards the other, resulting from an integration of loving and aggressive feelings. Partners identify with one another and are attuned to each other's radically different sexualities. There is mutual idealisation and commitment, and the relationship retains its passionate character. In his view, both man and woman wish the other to be man and woman for them, baby boy and baby girl, twin, soulmate, and adult sexual partner.

'*Le mariage est un duo ou un duel,*' I once read on a plaque above a mantelpiece. The duel is the married couple in which both partners attempt to be the answer to, or the question posed by, each other's lack. It is a mirror love that cannot tolerate difference, or where difference leads to endless (power) struggles. The duo, by contrast, is a couple that can tolerate a metaphorical third. A couple in which neither partner claims to be the other's solution, and both can leave each other in peace. If this form of mature love exists, it presupposes the renunciation of the doomed project of the ideal.

Notes

1 Gielkens, J., & Naaijkens, T. (1984). *Spiegel van de Duitse poëzie*. Amsterdam: Meulenhoff.
2 Bion, W. R. (1962/1984). *Learning from experience*. London: Karnac.
3 Soderbergh, S. (Director). (2002). *Solaris* [Film]. 20th Century Fox.
4 Russell, B. (1981). *De geschiedenis van de westerse filosofie*. Utrecht: Servire.
5 Lacan, J. (1964/1973). *Le Séminaire. Livre XI. Les quatre concepts fondamentaux de la psychanalyse*. Texte établi par J.A. Miller. Paris : Du Seuil.
6 Laroche-Parent, M. (1985). La femme (dite barrée) selon l'approche lacanienne. *Philosophiques*, *12*(1), 165–176.
7 De Botton, A. (1994). *Essays in love*. London: Picador.
8 My transl.: 'desire enhances things, but possession withers them'. Proust, M. (1896/2022). *Les Plaisirs et les Jours*. Paris: Calmann-Lévy.
9 Kernberg, O. F. (1998). *Love relations: Normality and pathology*. New Haven-London: Yale University Press.

12

Love Sung

Love and Poetry

When lovers declare their love to one another, their words inevitably take a metaphorical or allusive turn. Through love, they are, as it were, condemned to literature and sentenced to poetry. Love appears to trigger a full-blown factory of figurative expression. *L'amour, la poésie*, they seem symbiotically linked, as in the title of Paul Éluard's poetry collection.[1] It is certain that in love we are seized by something we do not understand. Nor can we say whether this something comes from within or without. It is as with the poet, who attributes his inspiration now to himself, now to his muse. In any case, both poet and lover attempt to capture this something in image and speech. They try to express and simultaneously contain the disruptive and dynamic force that love sets in motion. Even when love does not immediately strike like lightning, it invariably enacts a *coup d'état*.

Wherever Eros appears, both drive and the Thing are at play. They strike like a meteor, producing a burst of fireworks in our mental atmosphere. They pierce the brain's protective shell to touch our mind in special places – allegedly located somewhere in the amygdala. This is invariably accompanied by sensations nearly identical to those of fear. This fear, too, is the inextricable reverse of desire: fear of transgression, of self-loss, of total annihilation. On the way to a supposed fusion of apotheosis, all lovers become entangled in an alchemy of mutual identifications and a dizzying play of identities. Love is thus quintessentially a tale of 'the abyss and the airman' (Lucebert). It produces an imaginary deluge that floods everything, making thought drunk and reducing a few to drowning souls.

In one of her poems, Margaret Atwood calls mirrors perfect lovers.[2] Love oscillates between narcissism and idealisation. We mirror ourselves in the other, or we stand in adoration before that other. Narcissism is marked by a certain emptiness, by illusion and impossibility. Narcissus tries to touch his alluring reflection in the water, but '*Quod petis est nusquam*,' says Ovid in his *Metamorphoses*. 'What you seek is nowhere.' And only in this realisation lies liberation: '*Iste ergo sum! Sensi; nec me mea fallit imago*.'[3] 'So that is me. I know it. And the illusion deceives me no longer.' Unlike the narcissist, the lover does in fact have a (love-)object. The other may be idealised, but remains Other nonetheless.

DOI: 10.4324/9781003728764-13

Courtly Love

The historical connection between love and poetry reaches its peak with *courtoisie*.[4] This courtly love or *fin'amor* is a marvellous invention of the twelfth century – especially in southern France – the traces of which still resonate in today's rituals of courtship.

From a forward-looking perspective, courtly love is about unattainability. '*L'amour courtois est une sublimation, dans la mesure où il élève la femme à la dignité de la Chose'* – courtly love is a sublimation insofar as it elevates the woman to the dignity of the Thing.[5] This form of love, apart from any consummation, transforms itself into idealisation, servitude, and a blend of suffering and a sublime form of longing. The beloved lady transcends the Real and becomes a symbol of absence: a Thing that is desired but cannot be possessed. She thus nourishes an unfulfillable desire, arising from a void or lack that in turn drives her lover. Counterintuitively, this desire is sustained precisely by keeping the lady at a distance.

It is love as distilled perfection, as pure refinement, and as a form of art. Though essentially adulterous, it unfolds according to a precise (honour) code. The lady or *Domina* exerts a hold over the courtly lover, '*une saisie*. He becomes a 'servant of Eros'[6] and performs his service in a style characterised by noble bearing, avoidance of arrogance or vulgarity, a joyful and generous attitude, absolute respect for the woman, and last but not least, the secrecy of the (name of the) lady. This secrecy is the indispensable guarantee of her exaltation and perfection.

Unlike Platonic love, courtly love is consummated, but its primary realisation lies in incantation and courtly song. The voice of the troubadour, singing his love in *tempo rubato*, becomes emotion incarnate; his *joi* is ecstatic delight (*jouissance*, in Lacanian terms). The typical *canso* of, for example Arnaut Daniel, neither describes nor tells anything. It is its own message, a pure expression of amorous intensity. The lady is nothing more than an imaginary addressee, a mere pretext for his song.

At the manifest level, courtly song centres on the lady. But more fundamentally, she functions as a vessel of sound that envelops emptiness, making her the prototype of all art and sublimation. It is a love song whose *joi* stems from the abundance of meaning it generates. Various stylistic devices play a role here: the breaking open of syntax, lush paradoxes, the oxymoronic use of metaphor, and, more broadly, a libidinal engagement with language. Brimming with (oral) *jouissance*, the courtly singer stands at the 'balcony' of his lady. He revels in his own verbal mastery and hers alike, his tongue (*lalangue*) turning him into a kind of master of cunnilinguistics.

Prosaic

In the centuries that followed, song and poetry gradually drifted apart. Narrative began to emerge – initially in verse, later in prose. Satire supplanted idealisation, and the lyrical first-person gave way to the more epic third-person perspective.

The division wrought by language is captured in Jacques Lacan's distinction between the *sujet de l'énonciation* (the subject of the enunciation) and the *sujet de l'énoncé* (the subject of the statement). It is within this rift that the subject takes form.[7] When I begin a sentence with the word 'I' as its grammatical subject, the thinking Thing within me (Descartes' *res cogitans*)[8] vanishes beneath the fracture line of that 'I.' Cultural philosopher Marc De Kesel likens this phenomenon to Baron von Münchhausen pulling himself out of a swamp by his own hair.[9] Or to Felix the Cat, who, having overshot a bend, suddenly becomes aware of the abyss beneath him and, miraculously, propels himself back to solid ground from out of nothingness.

Keeping this opposition in mind, one might see the song as *énonciation* par excellence, and the narrative as *énoncé*. The song, in its act of saying, aims at subjective performance – it is emotion made flesh and given voice. Like love, it reasons without reason and is directed towards enjoyment. The story, by contrast, is concerned with what is said – targeting communication or instruction. Its reason is voiceless. It tends to banish love and enjoyment, along with the capacity for idealisation that underlies them. The reality principle assumes control, and gradually, a pact with reality is formed. Only with the advent of Romanticism, according to Julia Kristeva, is there any revival of courtly lyricism.[10] By then, the ideal takes on an impossible or fatal form, and emotionality presents itself as nostalgia – often as melancholy, but seldom again as *joi*. A loss of being has occurred; the original object can no longer be recovered in any manifold enthusiasm.

Heart of Darkness

According to Georges Bataille, love desires the impossible ('*la poésie veut l'impossible.*') The Good that was once symbolised by the lady becomes, after Baudelaire, more of an Evil (*le Mal*) a site of suffering and pleasure.[11] Passion springs from this as a blossoming of words: the painful and ecstatic language of his famous poetry collection *Les Fleurs du Mal*.[12] The view Baudelaire expresses in *Fusées* may be considered the dark counterpoint to courtly love: '*La volupté unique et suprême de l'amour gît dans la certitude de faire le mal*' – 'The unique and supreme voluptuousness of love lies in the certainty of doing evil.'

According to Milan Kundera, the art of the novel was born of God's laughter.[13] In his essays of the same name (which he tellingly refers to as the confessions of a practitioner), he links this moment to the birth of Greek philosophy, after which the 'passion for knowledge' took hold of humanity. As a deviation of this passion, the *Lebenswelt* – the lived world – would be increasingly excluded from technological and scientific inquiry. This derailment is sometimes referred to as the 'forgetting of Being.'[14] For Kundera, knowledge is the only morality of the novel. The novel is a unique exploration of the unknown parts of existence – without ever eclipsing its existential relativity and ambiguity. The spirit of the novel is the spirit of complexity and, as such, excludes totalitarian claims to truth. Poetry and philosophy ('the art of reason') cannot integrate the novel, but the reverse is possible. The only reason for the novel to exist is to say what only the novel can say. The novelist is a seismograph of his time. He is neither historian nor prophet, but an explorer of existence. Through his characters – 'experimental egos' – he investigates the possibilities of the human being in the trap that life has become.

Bleak

It may sound a little bleak, but in this light, prose might well be frustrated poetry. Every cynic is a disappointed romantic. One thinks of the distinction Kundera makes in *The Unbearable Lightness of Being* between the lyrical and the epic womaniser.[15] The former searches in every woman for his ideal; the latter sets out to explore the infinite diversity offered by the realm of Woman.

According to Simone de Beauvoir, no essence can define women once and for all.[16] Their sex, as it were, punches a hole in the symbolic order. Lacan argues that courtly love offers a symbolic buffer against the traumatic Real of desire and sexuality. By structuring love so that it is never fulfilled, the subject remains safe within the domain of symbolic and imaginary projection. Courtly love thus creates a form of controlled distance from *jouissance*, wherein tension persists but the threat of the Real never fully materialises.

As Gustave Courbet's famous painting suggests, this hole of the Real is *L'Origine du Monde,*[17] the origin of the world. Or, as the chansonnier Léo Ferré sings, '*Cette blessure d'où je viens'* – the wound from which I come.[18] We may try to defend ourselves against it through an imaginary hypertrophy of language, but against this jungle patch, neither poetic condensation nor prosaic displacement can prevail.

Notes

1 Eluard, P. (1929/2023). *L'amour la poésie*. Paris: République Lett.
2 Atwood, M. (1976). *Selected poems*. New York: Simon and Schuster.
3 Ovidius. (1976). *Metamorphoses*. London: Heinemann Loeb Classical Library.
4 Bec, P. (1992). *Écrits sur les troubadours et la lyrique médiévale*. Paris: Ed Paradigme.
5 Lacan, J. (1959–1960/1986). *Le Séminaire. Livre VII. L'éthique de la psychanalyse* (p. 152). Texte établi J-A. Miller. Paris: Seuil.
6 A memorable expression by Coetzee, J. M. (1999). *Disgrace*. New York: Vintage.
7 Lacan, J. (2001). *Autres écrits* (p. 426). Paris: Seuil.
8 Descartes, R. (1641/1989). *Meditaties*. Amsterdam/Meppel: Boom.
9 De Kesel, M. (2002). *Eros en Ethiek*. Leuven/Leusden: Acco.
10 Kristeva, J. (1985). *Histoires d'amour*. Paris: Gallimard.
11 Bataille, G. (1957). *L'érotisme*. Paris: Minuit.
12 Baudelaire, C. (1887/1986). Fusées. *Mon cœur mis à nu. La Belgique déshabillée*. Paris: Flammarion.
13 Kundera, M. (1986). *De kunst van de roman*. Amsterdam: Ambo.
14 Mayer, V. (2020). *Edmund Husserl, denken zonder oordelen*. Amsterdam: Abraxas|Zuider-Amstelboeken.
15 Kundera, M. (1985). *De ondraaglijke lichtheid van het bestaan*. Amsterdam: Ambo.
16 De Beauvoir, S. (1947/1986). *Le deuxième sexe*. Paris: Gallimard.
17 Courbet, G. (1866). *L'Origine du monde [Olieverf op doek]*. Paris: Musée d'Orsay. The painting was purchased in 1955 by Jacques Lacan. Because Lacan feared that the work was too fragile and too shocking to simply hang on the wall of his apartment, he had it built into a wooden sliding panel (a cache) painted by André Masson. See Didi-Huberman, G. (1999). *L'Origine du monde* de Courbet. Paris : Gallimard.
18 Ferré, L. (1970). Cette Blessure. *Amour Anarchie* (Vol. 2). Barclay Records. Paris.

13

Artful Love

Beauty

With palpable melancholy, Ludwig Vandevelde once created a sculpture in which a few words were scattered. When pieced together, they formed the question: *Dites-moi, où est-elle, la Beauté?* – 'Tell me, where is Beauty?'[1] As though beauty had entirely vanished from contemporary art, and we were now witnessing a peak era of the abject. In my memory, it involved a dismembered female body. I found it erotic and melancholic at once. Decades later, when I looked up the work, it turned out to depict a giant ear, laid open alongside its inner structures. Memory is deceptive. I had perhaps transformed it into a female body, given its rounded shapes and the use of black-stained oak. The body of Mother Woman is, after all, the first landscape we encounter in life, and the Imaginary register that also governs poetry is closely bound to our – her – body image. There also hangs a black ear on a black cardboard background by Yves Velter in my consulting room. It fits in perfectly; from a professional standpoint, the ear is by far my most active organ. If one tries to observe it 'objectively' – like an alien might – then it is ugly and repulsive. The Gestalt, or image, shields us from visceral ugliness, just as every skin hides much filth. This Imaginary register is one we share with animals. In mimicry, it allows them to merge with their environment, chameleon-like. In courtship, it is essential to display.

Psychoanalytically speaking, physical beauty can arouse both desire and paralysis. For Jacques Lacan, it cloaks or disguises the truth.[2] This resonates with a famous line from Rainer Maria Rilke's *First Duino Elegy*: *Das Schöne ist nichts als des Schrecklichen Anfang* – beauty is nothing but the beginning of terror.[3] The fragrant truth of cunnilingus, for instance, is veiled by feminine beauty.[4] Deep down, many men cannot handle the horror of the Real, i.e. castration. They have little taste for the details of female anatomy. Beauty may suspend their desire. It disarms, intimidates.[5]

Beautiful forms may inspire love and respect, but they can mute the drive. A beautiful woman on one's arm is a dazzling trophy, a phallic symbol for the hunter. Yet the ideal woman remains more of a loving, self-sacrificing mother 1 than a desiring or desirable mother 2. The man places her on a pedestal and turns her into

DOI: 10.4324/9781003728764-14

a Lady or goddess rather than confronting the wetness of her desire. For Stendhal, the ideal woman still had to be a '*âme sublime*' (a sublime soul).[6] In contemporary media, she appears as a pale, anorexic, androgynous ephebe. Her eroticism is at best auto-erotic: when she pouts, it seems she is kissing herself.

Sublimation

According to Freud, sublimation is the process by which sexual energy is diverted from its sexual aim to become a driving force behind cultural achievements such as art, science, and so forth. For Lacan, sublimation is less about changing the aim than about changing the object. Not only the drive, but also the beloved, is sublimated. Lacan elevates courtly love – or *fin'amor* – to the paradigm of sublimation.[7] It is the *fin'amor* with its exaltation of the woman and its cult of the idealised or sublimated beloved. In courtly love, the opposite sex is wrapped in narcissism, made untouchable, and encircled by an insurmountable linguistic barrier. A peculiar barrier, to be sure: for the troubadour attempts simultaneously to install and to overcome it through his songs of courtship. And all this for a Lady who may, like the muse, be nothing more than the projected feminine half of his own soul. We recall a few lines from Shakespeare's 34th sonnet: *What can mine own praise to mine own self bring/And what is 't but my own when I praise thee?*[8]

By placing obstacles in the path of sexual fulfilment, passion is intensified, and infatuation is amplified. *Make love* (literally: to create love) is, for Lacan, a creative process involving a shift from the Real to the Symbolic. A leap is made from the man who merely takes what he wants to the man who longs to be desired by the woman and aims to conquer the desire of the Big Other. In a striking definition of sublimation, the (love/art) object is elevated to the dignity of the Thing.[9]

Before the emergence of this form of love, relationships were based on lust and possession. The man was the owner of both the woman and the children. Especially within the upper classes, women were not considered human beings but rather objects of exchange – signifiers to be symbolically traded.[10] It was precisely these men who began to appreciate courtly lyricism.[11] In its elementary form, this concerns a knight courting his Lord's Lady. There is a double betrayal at play: that of the Lady and that of the knight or young lord towards their older Lord. In other words, we are dealing with a quasi-Oedipal rivalry, theatrically staged in the triangular relationship between Tristan, King Mark, and Isolde.

Courtly Love

Lacan speaks ironically of the *scholasticism of unhappy love*, in which the love object is cultivated in advance as a lost object over which the lover mourns.[12] Tellingly, the two never reach the passionate rhythms of a salsa or a tango – at best, they move in the slow, circling steps of a farewell waltz. In courtly culture, it is not the feeling itself that matters most, but the stylisation and aesthetic rendering of that feeling. The hallmark of courtly love lies not in authenticity, but in the degree of artistry with which the longing for the unapproachable Lady is expressed. It is more a matter of art than of love. At its centre lies an artificial construct, which, upon closer inspection, reveals itself to be highly unreal. The Lady makes a hollow, stereotypical impression. Though dazzling, she sets the heart ablaze, yet her beauty remains an irremovable veil. Courtly love appears faithful due to its noble selflessness and willingness to sacrifice. But what does this loyalty truly mean, when in the end the courtly lover and his (often older, married) Lady are not even bound together in lawful union?

Denis de Rougemont linked the rise of Romanticism to the spread of courtly love.[13] For him, the romantic relationship is not a universal given but a relatively recent and specifically Western invention. It begins with the troubadours and continues through *La Nouvelle Héloïse* (Julie, or the New Heloise) by Jean-Jacques Rousseau[14] and Goethe's *Die Leiden des Jungen Werthers* (The Sorrows of Young Werther).[15] In Romanticism, words not only describe feelings – they also evoke them. Rhetoric and eroticism become inextricably intertwined.

Artefact

Love takes a detour and becomes a work of art or artefact. It is a construction that redirects its course from physical to another kind of satisfaction. *Jouissance* is stirred: that paradoxical pleasurable displeasure which arises precisely through deferral or denial. The woman is catapulted into the stratosphere, and passion becomes – like *l'art pour l'art* – a passion for passion itself. The particularity of the woman is lost in this process of refinement, and the Lady in question is described time and again in the same stereotypical terms.[16]

Through the act of sublimation, man casts a kind of bait before himself – something he can yearn for and continue to desire. More broadly speaking, culture keeps us on the hook, holding out the promise of eventually fulfilling that desire. What binds us to our culture is precisely the transgressive space of fantasy, in which we may linger endlessly without danger to body or limb. This is, ultimately, the one true function of the Beautiful: that we may momentarily enter the domain of the Thing while not only preserving our subjectivity but even being able to develop it.

Desire and drive are analogous to Beauty and the Beast. Desire belongs to the (symbolic-imaginary) realm of the Big Other, while *jouissance* dwells more within the dark thrill of the Thing.[17]

Notes

1 Ludwig Vandevelde '*De l'esthétique*' Rijksmuseum Twenthe in Enschede. https://artfacts.net/exhibition/ludwig-vandevelde-de-l-esthetique-produzentengalerie-hamburg-hamburg-1991
2 Lacan, J. (1959–1960/1986). *Le Séminaire. Livre VII. L'éthique de la psychanalyse* (pp. 216–217). Texte établi par J. A. Miller. Paris: Seuil.
3 Rilke, R. M. (1922). *Duineser Elegien.* Berlin: Suhrkamp, 1975.
4 Lacan, J. (1959–1960/1986). *Le Séminaire. Livre VII. L'éthique de la psychanalyse* (p. 162). Texte établi par J. A. Miller. Paris: Seuil.

5 Lacan, J. (1959–1960/1986). *Le Séminaire. Livre VII. L'éthique de la psychanalyse* (p. 238). Texte établi par J. A. Miller. Paris: Seuil.
6 Stendhal. (1822/1980). *De l'amour* (p. 60). Paris: Gallimard.
7 Lacan, J. (1959–1960/1986). *Le Séminaire. Livre VII. L'éthique de la psychanalyse* (p. 162). Texte établi par J. A. Miller. Paris: Seuil.
8 Shakespeare, W. (1609/2008). *Sonnet 39*. In K. Duncan-Jones (Ed.), *Shakespeare's Sonnets* (pp. 112–113). London: Arden Shakespeare.
9 Lacan, J. (1959–1960/1986). *Le Séminaire. Livre VII. L'éthique de la psychanalyse* (p. 146). Texte établi par J. A. Miller. Paris: Seuil.
10 Lacan, J. (1959–1960/1986). *Le Séminaire. Livre VII. L'éthique de la psychanalyse* (pp. 214–215). Texte établi par J. A. Miller. Paris: Seuil.
11 Lacan, J. (1959–1960/1986). *Le Séminaire. Livre VII. L'éthique de la psychanalyse* (pp. 147–148). Texte établi par J. A. Miller. Paris: Seuil.
12 Lacan, J. (1959–1960/1986). *Le Séminaire. Livre VII. L'éthique de la psychanalyse* (pp. 147–148). Texte établi par J. A. Miller. Paris: Seuil.
13 De Rougemont, D. (1949). *Liefde en avondland*. Amsterdam: Uitgeversmaatschappij Holland.
14 Rousseau, J.-J. (1761/1993). *Julie, ou la Nouvelle Héloïse* (M. H. de la Roche, Ed.). Paris: Gallimard.
15 Goethe, J. W. von. (1774/1996). *Die Leiden des jungen Werthers* (H. Fröhlich, Hrsg.). Frankfurt am Main: Deutscher Klassiker Verlag.
16 Lacan, J. (1959–1960/1986). *Le Séminaire. Livre VII. L'éthique de la psychanalyse* (pp. 149–150). Texte établi par J. A. Miller. Paris: Seuil.
17 Lacan, J. (1966). *Ecrits* (p. 853). Paris: Seuil.

14

Mystic Love

Moving

Love, in its most radical form, exceeds the boundaries of psychology, biology, and culture. It *moves* us towards what lies beyond knowledge. Love has always been a mystical experience: it opens the subject to an Other that cannot be mastered, symbolised, or possessed. Psychoanalysis, though born from Enlightenment rationality,[1] has always circled this territory of the unsayable. We are reminded of Ludwig Wittgenstein: 'There is the inexpressible. This shows itself; it is the mystical.'[2] Mystic love in its narrow sense, on the other hand, has always stood at the threshold between theology and psychology, between transcendence and the unconscious. It evokes the longing for absolute union: the wish to lose oneself entirely in the beloved, in God, or in the Other. In modern psychoanalytic thought, such longing becomes a privileged site for exploring desire itself: not as fulfilment, but as the structure of human subjectivity. Two compatriot psychoanalysts have repeatedly published on this topic: Marc De Kesel[3] and Paul Moyaert.[4] In the religious overtones of mystic matters, I am rather amateurish myself, but this transcendental dimension of love can hardly be neglected, let alone dismissed. Therefore, I am very much indebted to their inspiration on these solemn affairs. On the other hand, I am more familiar with the mystical inclinations of Wilfred Bion, James Grotstein, and Michael Eigen.[5] Rudi Vermote once drew a distinction between Oedipus' conquering knowledge and the more intuitive openness to knowledge of the Sphinx.[6] I guess this binocular perspective can be very fruitful in psychoanalytic work. Also, on love.

Freud and Lacan

To begin with, Freud's suspicion of religion did not prevent him from recognising the force of mystical experience. In *Civilisation and Its Discontents*, he famously refers to the 'oceanic feeling' of boundless unity described by Romain Rolland, interpreting it as a regression to the infantile state of undifferentiated fusion with the mother.[7] For Freud, the mystical dissolution of boundaries signified not transcendence but a return to primary narcissism: the illusion of omnipotence

DOI: 10.4324/9781003728764-15

that precedes the formation of the ego. Yet, Freud's own theory of love, oscillating among need, demand, and desire, already hints at something irreducible to drive or ego. His view that all tenderness hides a trace of the sexual drive, and that every erotic tie bears the mark of loss, reveals a paradox: the drive towards union is inseparable from the experience of separation. Lacan would radicalise this paradox. In his reading of mysticism, particularly in Seminar XX: *Encore*, Lacan interprets the writings of female mystics, such as Teresa of Ávila, as testimonies to *jouissance*.[8] It is a form of enjoyment beyond pleasure, language, and the phallic economy. It arises when the subject momentarily brushes against the Real, that which cannot be symbolised or integrated. It is both union and rupture.

'God's love,' for Lacan, does not name a being but a limit: an encounter with the Real, where the subject experiences the impossibility of full knowledge.[9] The ecstatic union of the mystic does not close the gap between self and Other; it reveals it. Teresa's cry ('*Muero porque no muero*'/'I die because I do not die') expresses precisely this paradox of loving what cannot be possessed. Lacan sees in her writings an embodied metaphor for the structure of desire itself: to be ravished by what exceeds representation. Mystical love, then, is not a flight from the body but an intensification of embodiment. Teresa's trembling, her corporeal visions of divine arrows piercing the heart, were long dismissed as hysterical excess. Yet, from a psychoanalytic perspective, these experiences may reveal the body as the first site of the sacred, i.e. the stage upon which the drama of longing unfolds. Mysticism and psychoanalysis converge here: both explore the body's language as the theatre of the soul. Art provides an emblem of this ambiguity. Bernini's *Ecstasy of Saint Teresa*[10] captures a moment suspended between spiritual rapture and sensual arousal.[11] The saint's parted lips and arching body visualise the coincidence of divine and erotic pleasure. Psychoanalytically, this is not repression turned sacred but the revelation that sexual and mystical desires share a structure: both reach towards what cannot be possessed.

Erotic Religion

Marc De Kesel, therefore, argues that psychoanalysis's interest in mysticism does not stem from fascination with the experience of ecstasy, but with the *desire* for it.[12] Mysticism, especially in the Christian tradition, is saturated with *eros* – a yearning that can never be satisfied. Teresa of Ávila's cry expresses this endless tension: the desire to die to the self in order to live in God, yet the impossibility of completing that death.[13] What remains is the unfulfilled flame itself – *eros* purified of object, an ache that never ceases. De Kesel stresses this insight. For Freud, the human being is a *Wunschwesen* – a creature of wish and lack.[14] Desire, rather than the preservation of life, drives psychic life. In Lacan's reformulation, the subject is constituted by a void: the symbolic order fragments the unity of instinct, giving birth to the endless quest for the *objet petit a*, the missing fragment that can never be found. Mystical love and psychoanalytic desire thus converge: both revolve around absence.

To read mysticism as sublimated sexuality would be reductive. Yet, both operate through the same dynamic of lack. The mystic's longing for God is not a denial of the body but a transformation of its energies. In Lacanian terms, the desire is sexual because it is split (marked by loss and absence), not because it refers to intercourse. The *petite mort* of orgasm and the mystical death of the self are metaphors for a paradoxical survival through loss. Psychoanalysis illuminates this movement as a structural condition: the subject is always divided between the symbolic and the Real. Desire is thus the trace of an impossible reconciliation. Mystical love pushes this logic to its limit by seeking union with an infinite Other, only to discover an infinite separation.

Lacan famously called the primacy of desire the 'Copernican revolution' of psychoanalysis.[15] Instead of explaining desire through an antecedent fullness (paradise, nature, divine truth), psychoanalysis reverses the relation: such ideals exist only because desire produces them. Similarly, in the apophatic tradition of negative theology, the mystic must relinquish all images of God. The divine is unknowable, 'the dark night of the soul.'[16] In both cases, transcendence is redefined as absence.

Freud, too, approached this void when he wrote of religion as a collective neurosis, a projection of infantile wishes for protection and love.[17] Yet, the psychoanalytic critique does not destroy mysticism; it reveals its structural kinship with desire. The mystic's purification from idols parallels the analysand's traversal of fantasy. Both confront the lack that constitutes subjectivity.

Mystic love is not a relic of medieval piety but a persistent human pattern. In secular passion, the beloved often becomes a god-like figure, the mirror of one's ideal ego. Romantic literature, from Goethe's *Werther*[18] to Marguerite Duras' *L'Amant*,[19] stages this drama of excess and loss. Psychoanalytically, passion is a form of transference: the subject invests the other with the power to guarantee wholeness. When that illusion collapses, the subject confronts its constitutive lack once more. Freud saw in both religious devotion and erotic infatuation the same mechanism: displacement of infantile attachment onto new objects. Lacan radicalised this by interpreting love as the attempt 'to give what one does not have to someone who does not want it.' Love is thus an impossible exchange, grounded in absence. Mystic love is the purest form of love: it openly acknowledges that impossibility.

Complementary Perspectives

Donald Winnicott offers another way to approach mystical love. In *Playing and Reality*, he described the 'potential space' between inner and outer reality where creativity and illusion emerge.[20] Mystical experience, like play, inhabits this intermediate zone: it is neither hallucination nor objective encounter but a shared area of meaning. The mystic's language poetic, metaphorical, often erotic – serves to sustain this space of imaginative truth.

From a clinical perspective, such experiences can be integrative or regressive. When held within symbolic form – ritual, prayer, poetry – they can enrich psychic life. When severed from reality, they risk psychotic fusion or fanaticism.

Psychoanalysis thus seeks not to demystify mystic love but to contain it within language, where desire can circulate without consuming the self.

Contemporary research supports the view that mystical and romantic experiences share neural substrates. Beauregard and Paquette found that Carmelite nuns in prayer activated brain regions associated with both emotion and reward.[21] Helen Fisher identified similar dopaminergic circuits in romantic love.[22] These findings do not reduce spirituality to neurochemistry; rather, they show that the longing for transcendence is embodied. The psyche's metaphors are inscribed in the brain's pathways of pleasure and attachment.

Mystical and erotic love both court danger. The desire for dissolution can lead to obsession, dependence, or self-annihilation. Freud described the 'death drive' as the tendency to return to an inorganic state – a longing for quiescence beyond pleasure.[23] The mystic's yearning to 'die into God' borders on this drive. Yet, psychoanalysis reframes it as a quest for meaning within finitude. To desire absolutely is human; to survive desire is divine.

Clinically, mystic or passionate experiences can mask unresolved trauma. A patient repeatedly drawn to unavailable partners may be re-enacting the absence of a parental figure. Another may seek transcendence through meditation as an escape from depression. In both cases, analysis aims not to extinguish longing but to integrate it – to transform compulsive repetition into creative sublimation.

For Lacan, the ethical imperative of psychoanalysis is '*ne pas céder sur son désir*' – not to give up on one's desire. This does not mean pursuing satisfaction, but remaining faithful to the truth that desire reveals: our constitutive lack. Mystic love embodies this fidelity. Teresa's paradoxical joy in incompletion, Ruusbroec's language of *selfless use*, Rumi's celebration of longing as divine fire – all affirm desire as the path, not the obstacle.[24]

Mystic love and psychoanalysis meet in their confrontation with the impossible. Both reject the fantasy of total unity and instead cultivate an ethics of separation. The mystic's night of the soul and the analysand's encounter with the unconscious are parallel journeys through lack. What they discover is not the abolition of the self but its transformation through desire. As De Kesel writes, 'Mysticism deconstructs itself at the point where God disappears.'[25] The disappearance of the divine does not end love; it reveals love's structure: endless, ungrounded, creative. To love mystically is to accept the wound of desire as one's deepest truth.

Mystic love, then, is neither purely religious nor purely psychological. It is the name for that space where longing becomes thought, where absence becomes presence through language. Psychoanalysis, far from opposing mysticism, continues its work by other means: deciphering the divine within the human, the infinite within the lack.

Bion and Eigen

Where Freud saw regression, and Lacan saw the topology of the Real, Bion discerned a path of *faith*. In *Attention and Interpretation*, he speaks of the analyst's task as a discipline of 'negative capability,' echoing Keats's phrase for the capacity to dwell in uncertainty without reaching after fact or reason.[26] Bion introduces the concept of *O*: ultimate reality, the truth of experience that can never be known directly but only approached through a state of reverent openness.[27] To 'become O' is to surrender the ego's defences and allow the unknown to transform thought. Bion's mysticism is rigorous and secular: it demands an act of faith not in dogma but in the analytic process itself, where meaning arises from silence, not interpretation.

Michael Eigen extends this line of thought in *The Psychoanalytic Mystic*.[28] For Eigen, psychoanalysis at its best *is* a mystical discipline, a practice of love and faith in the face of psychic pain. The analytic relationship, like the mystical encounter, unfolds in a space of radical openness. It is what he calls the *terror of openness*, the capacity to feel life in its full intensity. He reinterprets Bion's *O* as an ever-present invitation to experience rather than to know. Analysis becomes an apprenticeship in devotion: to listen, to be moved, to remain porous to the suffering and vitality of the other. According to Eigen, psychoanalysis at its best becomes a mystical discipline, a work of faith and love, touching the unknown that lives through us.[29] In Eigen's universe, mysticism is not the negation of human affect but its deepest realisation. The analytic situation offers moments of grace: silences in which analyst and patient share an awareness of something vast, tender, and terrifying. Such moments cannot be manufactured; they emerge when both partners consent to not-knowing. The mystic's humility and the analyst's evenly suspended attention are twin forms of receptivity. They are a surrender to what Christopher Bollas might call the *unthought known*.[30] The mystical dimension of love is thus inseparable from vulnerability: to love is to expose oneself to annihilation and transformation alike.

Meister Eckhart, the medieval Dominican mystic, spoke of *Gelassenheit* (letting-be) as the path to union with the divine.[31] He taught that one must 'let God be God in us,' a process that requires the emptying of all images, including the image of God itself. This *via negativa* anticipates Bion's call to abandon memory and desire in the analytic session. Both Eckhart and Bion warn against the idolatry of certainty: only through unknowing can one encounter truth. Eckhart's insight that 'the eye with which I see God is the same eye with which God sees me' encapsulates the mutuality of mystical love. It is a reciprocity that mirrors the analytic dyad, where the subject discovers itself in the eyes, ears, heart, and mind of the other.

In the writings of Teresa of Ávila and Eckhart alike, divine love is an event of *kenosis*, of self-emptying.[32] The mystic's union is not a merger of substances but a meeting in absence. Similarly, the analyst's capacity to love the patient lies not in identification but in the disciplined creation of an empty space where psychic truth can appear. Love is not possession but hospitality: an opening through which the other may come to be. In this way, the psychoanalytic and the mystical share a grammar of waiting. Both cultivate a form of attention that is neither passive nor active, but receptive. It is a 'faith in waiting,' as Bion phrased it.[33] In such waiting, time suspends itself; what emerges is not revelation but relation. Love, as mystic and analyst alike discover, is less a feeling than a mode of being-with: a dwelling at the border of the known and the unknowable.

Notes

1 https://www.prospectmagazine.co.uk/culture/49771/freud-the-last-great-enlightenment-thinker

2 My transl. Wittgenstein, L. (1921/1999). *Tractatus logico-philosophicus* (W.F. Hermans Vert.). Amsterdam: Boom, Stelling 6.522.

3 De Kesel, M. (2017). *Zelfloos: De mystieke afgrond van het moderne ik.* Utrecht: Kok; De Kesel, M. (2021). *Ik, God & mezelf: Mystiek als deconstructie.* Amsterdam: Sjibbolet.

4 Moyaert, P. (1998). *De mateloosheid van het christendom: Over naastenliefde, betekenisincarnatie en mystieke liefde.* Nijmegen: SUN; Moyaert, P. (2002). Passie en mystieke liefde. In Thys, M. & Kinet, M. (Red.), *Liefdesverklaringen* (pp. 141–154). Leuven/Leusden: Acco.

5 Bion, W. R. (1970). *Attention and interpretation.* London: Tavistock Publications; Grotstein, J. S. (2007). *A beam of intense darkness: Wilfred Bion's legacy to psychoanalysis.* London: Karnac. Eigen, M. (1998). *The psychoanalytic mystic.* New York: Jason Aronson.

6 Vermote, R. (1994). Le mythe d'Oedipe à la lumière du Sphinx. *Revue Belge de Psychanalyse, 24*, 29–42.

7 Freud, S. (1930/1961). *Civilization and its discontents* (J. Strachey, Ed. & Trans.). London: Hogarth Press.

8 Lacan, J. (1972–1973/1998). *The seminar of Jacques Lacan, Book XX: Encore (On feminine sexuality, the limits of love and knowledge, 1972–1973)* (B. Fink, Trans.). New York: Norton.

9 Lacan, J. (1972–1973/1998). *The seminar of Jacques Lacan, Book XX: Encore (On feminine sexuality, the limits of love and knowledge, 1972–1973)* (B. Fink, Trans., pp. 69–74). New York: Norton.

10 Bernini, G. L. (1647–1652). *The ecstasy of Saint Teresa [Marble sculpture, Cornaro Chapel, Santa Maria della Vittoria, Rome, Italy].* In Hibbard, H. (1990). *Bernini* (pp. 158–160). London: Penguin Books.

11 Treffers, B. (1995). *Een hemel op aarde: Extase in de Romeinse barok.* Nijmegen: SUN.

12 De Kesel, M. (2017). *Zelfloos: De mystieke afgrond van het moderne ik.* Utrecht: Kok.

13 Teresia van Avila. (1577/1982). *Mystieke werken 3: Innerlijke burcht, gewetensbrieven, kleinere geschriften* (C. Noyen, Trans.). Gent: Carmelitana; Teresa of Ávila. (1565/1961). *The life of Saint Teresa of Ávila by herself* (J. M. Cohen, Trans.). London: Penguin Classics.

14 Freud, S. (1920/1955). Beyond the pleasure principle (J. Strachey, Trans.). In *The standard edition of the complete psychological works of Sigmund Freud* (Vol. 18, pp. 1–64). London: Hogarth Press.

15 Lacan, J. (1955/1966). La chose freudienne ou le sens du retour à Freud en psychanalyse. In *Écrits* (pp. 401–436, p. 418). Paris: Seuil.

16 John of the Cross. (1584/1991). *The spiritual canticle* (K. Kavanaugh & O. Rodriguez, Trans.). New York: Paulist Press.

17 Freud, S. (1921/1960). Group psychology and the analysis of the ego (J. Strachey, Trans.). In *The standard edition of the complete psychological works of Sigmund Freud* (Vol. 18, pp. 67–143). London: Hogarth Press.

18 Goethe, J. W. von. (1774/1989). *The sorrows of young Werther* (M. Hulse, Trans.). London: Penguin.

19 Duras, M. (1984). *L'amant.* Paris: Minuit.

20 Winnicott, D. W. (1971/2005). *Playing and reality.* London/New York: Routledge.

21 Beauregard, M., & Paquette, V. (2006). Neural correlates of a mystical experience in Carmelite nuns. *Neuroscience Letters, 405*(3), 186–190.

22 Fisher, H. E. (2004). *Why we love: The nature and chemistry of romantic love*. London: Henry Holt and Company.
23 Freud, S. (1920/1955). Beyond the pleasure principle (J. Strachey, Trans.). In *The standard edition of the complete psychological works of Sigmund Freud* (Vol. 18, pp. 1–64). London: Hogarth Press.
24 Rumi. (ca. 1250/1995). *The essential Rumi* (C. Barks, Trans.). New York: HarperCollins.
25 De Kesel, M. (2021). *Ik, God & mezelf: Mystiek als deconstructie*. Amsterdam: Sjibbolet.
26 Bion, W. R. (1970). *Attention and interpretation*. London: Tavistock Publications.
27 Bion, W. R. (1970). *Attention and interpretation* (p. 44). London: Tavistock Publications.
28 Eigen, M. (1998). *The psychoanalytic mystic*. New York: Jason Aronson.
29 Eigen, M. (1998). *The psychoanalytic mystic* (p. 7). New York: Jason Aronson.
30 Bollas, C. (1987). *The shadow of the object: Psychoanalysis of the unthought known*. New York: Columbia UP.
31 Meister Eckhart. (1290–1327/1981). *The essential sermons, commentaries, treatises, and defence* (E. Colledge & B. McGinn, Eds. & Trans.). New York: Paulist Press.
32 Even for an atheist, Simone Weil writes movingly on this kenosis. Mijn vert.: "Creation is an act of self-emptying, a kenosis, in which God, by withdrawing, gives existence to that which is other than Himself." Weil, S. (1963). *La pesanteur et la grâce* (pp. 43–47). Paris: Plon.
33 Bion, W. R. (1970). *Attention and interpretation* (pp. 124–126). London: Tavistock Publications.

15

Love as an Event

Critical

Philosophers often make use of the term 'Critique.' Think, for instance, of Kant's *Critique of Pure Reason* or *Critique of Practical Reason*.[1] This is not about a qualitative or normative judgment, such as beautiful or ugly, right or wrong, good or evil, but about the analysis of an underlying dynamic or structure. The subject of critique can be highly mundane, if not banal. The Slovenian philosopher and psychoanalyst Slavoj Žižek, for example, delights in critiquing Hollywood films precisely to expose profound truths.[2] With that same licence, let's imagine (and examine) an infatuated couple, freewheeling on a bike. The girl on the back of the bicycle is over the moon. She muses: 'When I open my eyes and look all around, everything's different and my heart starts to pound. I feel so strange. I don't know what to do, and when I ask why, the reason is you.' Or: 'You're inside my heart, deep in my soul. You've been there from the start. Since the day I fell for you. You are inside the dream that I want to pursue.' Or: 'I'm riding with you on your bike. You're going faster and faster now. I barely see the road ahead. Do I jump off or vow to cast my fears aside today and never walk away?'

These thoughts, expressed in would-be poetical language, describe what happens when one falls in love. It is often a chance encounter, but one that, to the person concerned, nonetheless appears necessary. It is a happening. It even *had* to happen! In retrospect, everything seems to have led up to this fall. By submitting to this event, you also subjectivise it: you become more yourself. You are seized by a (causal) force in which you seem to find your true self, one that henceforth alters all the coordinates of your life. Gradually, a shared cause arises, whereby the lovers freely choose each other with a mutual sense of necessity.

Event

To deepen this further, I shift the focus to two philosophers strongly influenced by Hegel and Lacan: Alain Badiou and Slavoj Žižek. In his magnum opus, Alain Badiou elaborates on the concept of the *event*, which in his thought acquires

DOI: 10.4324/9781003728764-16

ontological status.[3] Events, for Badiou, can take place within four domains: science (e.g., Galileo, Einstein), art (e.g., Picasso, Schoenberg), politics (e.g., the French Revolution, May 1968), or love (anywhere in the world, at any hour of the day). For Badiou, an event creates a rupture in knowledge. *Un événement est ce qui n'est pas dans le compte de la situation*[4] – an event is that which does not figure in the account of the situation. It belongs to no pre-existing system of understanding. It seems impossible, and yet it happens. It arises outside the logic of the 'situation' and cannot be deduced from what already exists. It is always and irreducibly singular. It produces an excess, and precisely in this surplus, a subject is constituted while simultaneously identifying with the new truth that the event initiates.[5]

The event is a precarious supplement: it disappears the moment it appears. It is a timeless interruption of the ordinary course of things, which can nonetheless have lasting consequences for what follows.[6] The event is immediately absorbed into the unfolding of life, and yet continues to carry itself forward. It is, in the words of Vladimir Jankélévitch, both a *je-ne-sais-quoi* and a *presque rien* – a kind of near-nothing.[7] The truth it speaks is heterogeneous to the dominant opinion or the opinion of those in power. It causes a rupture. Conversely, one can only escape this rupture by returning to the world of goods and interests – by breaking with the break that seized you. In fidelity to the event, the subject effectively severs ties with the habitual ways of thinking and acting. 'Love is like two dreamers dreaming the exact same dream,' sings Michael Franks. This shared dream forms both the foundation and the point of departure from which lovers begin to challenge the armies of reality. The couple gradually evolves from *falling* in love to *standing* in love.

After the Big Bang of the encounter, truth particles disperse across a shared universe. Love cuts across the most significant oppositions and deepest ruptures. The world is henceforth built not alone, but by two – on *la vérité sur le Deux* ('the truth of Two').[8] The ecstasy of the encounter gives way to a sustained construction. It is a resolute adventure, for true love triumphs over the obstacles it encounters. The declaration of love marks the transition from encounter to the construction of truth. What began as a chance becomes the shared assumption of a new beginning.

For Badiou, love is a transformative experience that moves us beyond egocentrism and compels us to view the world from the perspective of the Other. In particular, in *In Praise of Love*, he presents a further philosophical defence of this conception of love against contemporary efforts to reduce it to convenience, safety, or contractual arrangements. Instead, he defines love as a radical process of truth-production. In his work, it becomes clear that love is not just about romantic feelings or physical attraction, but about creating a new truth that reshapes the lovers' shared reality.

Once, many years ago, I believed love meant finally being understood. Not agreed with – understood. It took me a long time to discover that understanding does not sustain love. Staying is.

Truth

Badiou regards love (alongside art, science, and politics) as one of the four truth procedures. This means that love is not simply a feeling or subjective experience, but a disruptive process – a means of bringing a new, shared truth into the world and thereby altering our perception of reality. Together, the lovers create a universe unique to their relationship, independent of the outside world and of the social norms that might otherwise restrict their existence.[9] Love begins from a chance encounter, but through a kind of act of faith, it invests in that encounter and remains faithful to it: *L'amour est ce qui fait confiance au hasard.*[10] Love is that which trusts in chance.

The great mystery of love, according to Badiou, lies in its ability to transform contingency into proof of truth. Love becomes a lasting construction. The declaration 'I love you' means: to fix the accidental in a timeless moment. *Tout amour se déclare éternel.*[11] Every love declares itself eternal. The fidelity that follows is a prolonged triumph over the fleeting nature of the encounter. All of this requires a form of existential courage: the willingness to open oneself up and to make something of the encounter, even when its outcome remains uncertain.

Contrary to rose-tinted or consumer-oriented notions of love, Badiou insists that love is a long-term process. True love is not merely the moment of falling in love, but the continuous work of building a shared world based on a life-model that is more than the sum of its individual parts.[12] This demands commitment, perseverance, and fidelity to the event. It is not simply a pleasurable experience, but also a struggle against obstacles and differences, in which the couple resists the (neoliberal) logic of instant gratification.[13] Badiou opposes the contemporary trend to frame love as a risk-free experience (such as dating apps that algorithmically match partners based on preferences and compatibility). He critiques this 'insurance logic' of love, where danger and pain are to be avoided at all costs. For him, love is valuable precisely because it is such an unpredictable undertaking. It presupposes a durable recognition – even embrace – of difference. Whereas sexual desire is often (fetishistically) directed towards part-objects such as breasts, buttocks, shoulders or penis, love is oriented towards the being of the other – an encounter that disrupts my own existence and reshapes it anew.[14]

Catastrophe

Badiou's perspective is ultimately affirmative – his title does not lie: it is a *praise* of love. Slavoj Žižek largely shares Badiou's orientation, yet his account of love is more traumatic and destabilising.[15] For Žižek, love is not a peaceful unification of two souls, but rather a radical interruption of the self. He argues that prior to love, we live in a kind of narcissistic self-sufficiency. Love comes as a shock that violently pulls us out of our egotism. One's world is suddenly reorganised around the Other, bringing anxiety, uncertainty, and vulnerability. Love is not healing – it does not fulfil us but instead confronts us with a lack we were reluctant to acknowledge.

It is a violent existential force that disrupts the symbolic order. It presupposes a leap into the unknown and compels us to redefine the self.

With this, Žižek builds on Lacan's famous *dictum*: *Aimer, c'est donner ce qu'on n'a pas à quelqu'un qui n'en veut pas.*[16] 'To love is to give what one does not have to someone who does not want it.' This suggests that love is not about possessing the other or finding a perfect match. Rather, love is about recognising – and even embracing – what is missing. These views directly challenge the 'Tinderification' of love, in which it is rationalised and filtered. The beloved is not a commodity whose qualities can be ticked off on a list. True love is at once subversive, chaotic, and unpredictable.

Like Badiou, Žižek criticises any conception of love as a contract or transaction in which one seeks a 'perfect' product. Instead, he describes love as a dialectical process in which the subject rediscovers itself through the encounter with the Other.[17] Love becomes a political act – it breaks through the hegemony of the polished, consumption-driven capitalist logic. For Žižek, love is not a romantic paradise but a catastrophe: it is the experience that confronts us with our own limitations and insufficiencies, pulling us out of our comfort zones and compelling us to recognise the Other not as an object of gratification but as a radical alterity.[18]

Let me return briefly to the bicycle's grounded realism for a typical love event. Imagine: you're at a party. You don't really know anyone; you chat a bit, drink something – everything feels familiar and predictable. Then, suddenly, you meet someone. You can't articulate why this particular encounter would be different, but it feels as if something fundamental is happening. *L'événement est l'impensable de la situation, son excès.*[19] The event is the unthinkable of the situation, its excess. Your view on life shifts. Not because this person solves everything, but because you suddenly realise: the world is no longer the same now that I know you exist. The Other breaks into your 'situation' – your habitual way of being, thinking, and feeling – without warning. When you choose to believe in this encounter, you begin a trajectory whose destination remains unknown, but to which you commit in the attempt to realise it.

Accident?

From Lacan to Žižek to Badiou, love is decidedly not viewed as a state of natural harmony. Gone is the ideal of romantic fusion or self-evident unity. Love arises from rupture, from lack, from the gap. For Lacan, love revolves around the linguistic lack of the symbolic order. We love in the Other something that reminds us of our own absence, and love becomes a form of misrecognition. It is inevitably marked by illusion, projection, and fantasy. It touches on – and simultaneously overshoots the Real. Love both reveals and conceals the lack. *Il n'y a pas de rapport sexuel*[20] – there is no such thing as a 'natural' sexual relation in human terms. *Et l'amour, c'est toujours ça: tenter de recoller le sujet à son manque.*[21] love is always this – an attempt to bind the subject to its lack. But that never entirely succeeds. Love, then, is a way of dealing with the fundamental void.

For Badiou, love is rooted in an event that disrupts the 'situation.' It is not misrecognition or illusion, but a constructive engagement. It opens up a new way of being-together-in-the-world – a truth-process that can never be predetermined. Žižek positions himself somewhere between the two. Personally, I would take my seat on the back of Žižek's bicycle, but I would try to keep my eyes open. Depending on the 'situation' and your sense of balance, the line between an *event* and an *accident* is often perilously thin…

Notes

1 De Boer, K. (2009). Kant, Hegel, en het begrip 'immanente kritiek' in de moderne filosofie. *Tijdschrift voor Filosofie, 71*(3), 475–498.
2 Žižek, S. (1992). *Looking awry: An introduction to Jacques Lacan through popular culture*. Cambridge: MIT Press.
3 Badiou, A. (1988). *L'être et l'événément*. Paris: Seuil.
4 Badiou, A. (1988). *L'être et l'événément* (p. 190). Paris: Seuil.
5 Badiou, A. (1988). *L'être et l'événément* (p. 192). Paris: Seuil.
6 Thys, M. (2024). Het avontuur van de psychoanalytische schriftuur. *Tijdschrift voor Psychoanalyse & haar toepassingen, 30*(3), 136–143.
7 Jankélévitch, V. (2014). *Le je-ne-sais-quoi et le presque-rien. La méconnaissance, le malentendu*. Paris: Seuil.
8 Badiou, A. (2009). Éloge *de l'amour* (p. 52). Paris: Flammarion.
9 Badiou, A. (2009). Éloge *de l'amour* (p. 52). Paris: Flammarion.
10 Badiou, A. (2009). Éloge *de l'amour* (p. 64). Paris: Flammarion.
11 Badiou, A. (2009). Éloge *de l'amour* (p. 72). Paris: Flammarion.
12 Badiou, A. (2008). *The concept of model* (Orig. *Le concept de modèle*). London/New York: Verso.
13 Badiou, A. (2012). *The rebirth of history: Times of riots and uprisings*. London/New York: Verso.
14 Roth, M. (2018). True love as the love of truth. *Psychoanalytic Perspectives, 15*, 190.
15 Žižek, S. (2008). *The fragile absolute – Or, why is the Christian legacy worth fighting for*. London/New York: Verso.
16 Lacan, J. (1960–1961/1991). *Le Séminaire. Livre VIII. Le transfert*. Texte établi par Jacques-Alain Miller (p. 143). Paris: Seuil.
17 Žižek, S. (2012). *Less than nothing: Hegel and the shadow of dialectical materialism*. London/New York: Verso.
18 Žižek, S. (2017). *Incontinence of the void: Economico-philosophical spandrels*. Cambridge: MITPress.
19 Badiou, A. (1988). *L'être et l'événément* (p. 192). Paris: Seuil.
20 Lacan, J. (1972–1973/1975). *Le Séminaire Livre XX. Encore*. Texte établi par Jacques-Alain Miller (p. 45). Paris: Seuil.
21 Lacan, J. (1972–1973/1975). *Le Séminaire Livre XX. Encore*. Texte établi par Jacques-Alain Miller (p. 13). Paris: Seuil.

16

The Beloved Mirror

Reflection

I see myself—
a silver eagle soaring high,
with cloud-tail wisps
like ribbons in the sky.
Above, the light and shadow blend,
a meteor's touch,
a flare, a bend.
And higher still—
I see myself
a lattice spun
of starlit wealth,
a sieve of light.
Like lanterns cast
in rippling water,
drifting past.
And there again—
myself I find,
a dolphin diving,
flickering, blind,
a trembling leap
towards a frog,
across some dream-lit
evening fog.
And there—reflected
in the glass,
beside which I,
carefree, lie back,

DOI: 10.4324/9781003728764-17

eyes turned upward,
soft and slow—
I see myself
in skyward glow.

I begin with this youthful poem to speak of the beloved as a mirror. There are other animals that can recognise themselves in a reflection, but according to Jacques Lacan, this sight evokes jubilation only in the human infant, an experience he considered fundamental.[1] While chimpanzees may play with their reflection, they are not captivated by it.[2] In this context, Lacan employs the term *Gestalt*. The still-fragmented and incoherent child sees itself, for the first time, as a whole in the mirror. This image serves as an anchoring point, but it is deceptive, as it contrasts with the actual experience of fragmentation and lack of coordination. Left and right, foreground and background, are not only distorted but even reversed. Try cutting your own hair in front of a mirror!

Gestalt

The mirror also idealises the body image. It presents us with an idealised version of ourselves – one we can only approach asymptotically, for we never truly become whole men or women.

The mirror image is an Ideal-Ego and forms a matrix in which the ego takes shape.[3] It provides an initial (imaginary) identification on which subsequent identifications gradually sediment. In essence, and following Arthur Rimbaud: *Je est un autre*.[4] Lacan calls this the mental disorder of the human, for the self is a problematic yet necessary fiction.[5] The ego is founded on *méconnaissance* – misrecognition – or *wishful seeing*: I see myself as I would like to be, flawless and complete. It is a form of identification but also of alienation, in which the ego arises from a leap of disarray (*désarroi*) towards an anticipated wholeness.[6] Compare it to the proclamation of a unified Germany long before any actual social, cultural, or economic unity had been achieved. The image functions as a prosthesis, enabling further development.

Drawing on film footage of children in front of mirrors, Lacan, in his eighth seminar, shows not only that the mirror image becomes libidinally invested but also how it is internalised or ratified through parental recognition.[7] Their words ('You are…') serve as primary signifiers that form the basis of the Ideal-Ego and, by extension, the core of later psychological identity.

Whereas primary narcissism is sometimes considered a kind of hardwired animal narcissism, for Lacan, it involves a far more complex operation. His concern is not with the narcissism of the biological organism prioritising self-preservation, but with that of the psychological subject. The imaginary register we share with animals is, in humans, restructured and overwritten by the symbolic order introduced by parental figures, who articulate their vision of the child.[8] The Ideal-Ego that results is not an imaginary projection but a symbolic introjection[9] – imposed from without by caregivers who see in us, or expect from us, something we can never fully attain.[10]

Freud initially sought the roots of love in infantile sexuality and the Oedipus complex, but with the introduction of narcissism, he took a different path.[11] Love then becomes a transfer of self-love or ego-libido to other objects (*'égaux'*). Libido flows from the self to the other, and when love fades or ends, the libido returns to the self. The beloved is chosen either out of need – resembling those who once met our needs – or by likeness, based on a pre-existing (unconscious) ideal. In both cases, the other becomes everything, and the self nothing. That is why Lacan calls love a form of suicide.[12]

The Imaginary

Lacan's renowned *retour à Freud* unfolded in three phases, evolving across his three registers: from the Imaginary to the Symbolic and back to the Real. The term 'Imaginary' primarily refers not to illusion, but to the structuring power of images. In his writings on the mirror stage and on aggressivity in psychoanalysis, Lacan draws on experimental psychology, optics, anthropology, and ethology.[13] He highlights the formative role images play in shaping developmental processes in animals.[14] A locust transforms as soon as it sees another of its kind. A female dove reaches sexual maturity upon perceiving the image of another dove.

The Imaginary is also central to aggressive behaviour. Ethologist Konrad Lorenz had already noted that animals are often more aggressive towards members of their own species than towards others.[15] Dominant and submissive postures have been observed in many species and are crucial for hierarchy and pecking order. The baring of teeth in a smile, for example may serve to indicate fear and to signal no intention of attack.[16] In the Imaginary, size does matter. The other (of the same species) is smaller, larger, stronger, or weaker – and also operates on the basis of the same premises. The Imaginary is fundamentally mimetic: one interprets the other's motives only through one's own drives. There is no recognition of the other *as* other, nor of what one does *to* the other. This Imaginary register dominates the animal kingdom, but also prevails in the earliest stages of human life.

Both animal pups and children can play together, but they are also often in fierce competition for the same parental resources. Few conflicts are as hateful or intense as those between siblings.[17] I refer to a pithy line by drive-theorist Leopold Szondi: *Kain regiert die Welt* ('Cain rules the world.').[18] The Imaginary also plays a leading role in courtship and mating displays. The peacock's tail and the nightingale's song are ostentatious advertisements of genetic value, and help determine their ranking in the sexual parade.

The Imaginary register is at its peak when relationships are chiefly marked by rivalry, power, and aggression, for it is only within the Symbolic register that ideals, authority, laws, rules, boundaries, and guilt begin to take precedence. In the consulting room, the psychoanalyst risks becoming trapped in the Imaginary when they take the patient's positive or negative feelings too personally, rather than interpreting them as transference. Lacan coined the neologism *hainamoration* (a blend of hatred, love, and adoration) to capture the dual nature of the Imaginary. For him, this is the very snare by which the analyst may be undone.[19]

Assault

This entire excursion through the Imaginary and (its relation to) narcissism is necessary to expose a self-centred dimension of love. When we seek fusion with the beloved, it is because we wish to rewind the clock: to a time before alienation and separation. We long to reunite with the 'lost half' from whom we were severed by Zeus, and thus attempt to undo an original loss. We perceive the other as a twin soul or soulmate. Certain declarations are characteristic: 'We are the same,' or 'We were made/born for each other.' The symbolic dimension of desire has then given way to the Imaginary dimension of passion.

As Sören Kierkegaard already noted, every passion presupposes the unconditional exclusion of a third party. Narcissism plays an essential role, for it is precisely the mutual resemblance through which lovers distinguish themselves from others that constitutes the core of infatuation.[20] In a typical pun, Lacan remarks: *ils se mêment dans l'autre* – they merge in the other. They love one another as similars, and they love themselves in the other.[21]

I close this beloved mirror with a question. Why are we drawn to creatures that are self-sufficient, like a tomcat or a beautiful man or woman? Is it because they seem sexually inaccessible and unattainable – or because they appear to possess a surplus of narcissism, from which we might share in their stardom? An *anaclitic* partner choice holds the promise of real, tangible satisfaction. The narcissistic one offers rather the prospect of (supposedly) Imaginary gratification. It is more *Mirage* than substance: not coincidentally, a synonym for both a *fata morgana* and the famed fighter jet by France's *Dassault*.

Notes

1 Narcissus is aware that the water shows his reflection and not some water spirit, see Ovidius. (1976). *Metamorphoses* (Vol. III, p. 350). London: Heinemann Loeb Classical Library.
2 Lacan, J. (1949/1966). Le stade du miroir comme formateur de la fonction du Je. In *Ecrits* (p. 93). Paris: Seuil.
3 Not the ego as a psychic apparatus from Freud's structural model, but rather the specular ego or the ego as self, as specifically understood by Lacan. See Kohut, H. (1971). *The analysis of the self.* New York: International UP.
4 Rimbaud, A. (1871/2006). Lettre du voyant/brief van de ziener aan Demeny (d.d. /05/1871). In *Ik is een ander, zienersbrieven, een seizoen in de hel en Illuminations* (H. Van Pinxteren, Vert.). Amsterdam: Veen.
5 Lacan, J. (1953–1954/1988). *The seminar of Jacques Lacan, Book I: Freud's papers on technique* (p. 16). New York: Norton.
6 Lacan, J. (1960–1961/1991). *Le Séminaire. Livre VIII. Le transfert* (J. A. Miller, Ed.). Paris: Seuil.

7 Lacan, J. (1960–1961/1991). *Le Séminaire. Livre VIII. Le transfert* (J. A. Miller, Ed.). Paris: Seuil.
8 Lacan, J. (1955–1956/1993). *The seminar of Jacques Lacan, book III: The psychoses* (J. A. Miller, Ed. & R. Grigg, Transl., p. 9). New York: Norton.
9 Lacan, J. (1957–1958/1998). *Le séminaire de Jacques Lacan, Livre V : Les formations de l'inconscient* (J. A. Miller, Ed., p. 402). Paris: Seuil.
10 Freud, S. (1914). On narcissism. In *Freud standard edition* (Vol. 14, p. 100). London: Hogarth.
11 Freud, S. (1914). On narcissism. In *Freud standard edition* (Vol. 14, p. 100). London: Hogarth.
12 Lacan, J. (1953–1954/1988). *The seminar of Jacques Lacan, Book I: Freud's papers on technique* (p. 149). New York: Norton.
13 Lacan, J. (1949/1966). Le stade du miroir comme formateur de la fonction du Je. In *Ecrits* (p. 93). Paris: Seuil.
14 Lacan, J. (2013). *On the names-of-the-father* (B. Fink, Transl., p. 12). Cambridge: Polity.
15 Lorenz, K. (1966). *On aggression* (Marjorie K. Wilson, Transl., p. 15). New York: Harcourt.
16 De Waal, F., & Tyack, P. L. (Eds.). (2003). *Animal social complexity: Intelligence, culture and indivdualized societies* (p. 278). Cambridge: Harvard University Press.
17 Sulloway, F. J. (1996). *Born to rebel: Birth order, family dynamics and creative lives.* New York: Pantheon.
18 Kinet, M. (2010). Pathoanalyse en antropopsychiatrie Het levenswerk van Jacques Schotte. *Tijdschrift voor Psychoanalyse, 3,* 191–197.
19 Lacan, J. (1960–1961/2015). *The seminar of Jacques Lacan, book VIII: Transference* (J. A. Miller & J. Forrester, Transl., p. 185). Cambridge: Polity.
20 Kierkegaard. (1847/1995). *Works of love* (H. V. Hong & E. H. Hong, Eds. & Transl., p. 50 en 56). Princeton: Princeton University Press.
21 Lacan, J. (1953–1954/1988). *The seminar of Jacques Lacan, Book I: Freud's papers on technique* (p. 85). New York: Norton.

Panoramic Intermezzo II

Once desire has awakened, it seeks forms.
It sings.
It paints.
It prays.
It thinks.

In this second movement, love leaves the intimate sphere and enters the cultural sphere.
It becomes an ideal, an artwork, a mysticism, an event, or a mirror.
Not because the human being escapes from reality, but because reality becomes uninhabitable without these forms.
The beloved is elevated; the voice becomes song; the touch becomes ritual; the encounter becomes an experience of truth.

What becomes evident here is how love continually transforms itself.
It seeks the absolute, yet can only speak in images.
It seeks unity, yet lives with fault lines.

In poetry, art and mysticism, love does not become greater than it is, but more precise: it reveals its paradoxical core — the longing for the impossible, lived within the possible.

The human being mirrors itself in the beloved and, at the same time, discovers that it never coincides with that image.

Thus love becomes at once exaltation and estrangement, revelation and illusion.
Not despite this tension, but because of it, love remains in motion.

DOI: 10.4324/9781003728764-18

17

Transference Love

Histoire d'O

What happens to love in the consulting room? One of Freud's most brilliant discoveries is arguably the phenomenon of transference. He initially encountered it indirectly, in its most spectacular and erotic form.[1] During their collaborative *Studies on Hysteria*, Freud's early mentor, Joseph Breuer, became entangled in the increasingly amorous feelings of his patient, Anna O.[2] Eventually, he visited her daily, sometimes for hours at a time. When his wife began to protest, and Breuer decided to terminate the treatment, the situation culminated in a hysterical pseudo-pregnancy. During her 'labour,' Anna O. famously exclaimed: 'Dr B's baby is on the way!'[3] This development led the poor Breuer to flee with his wife on a second honeymoon to Venice.[4]

Although Breuer's treatment of Anna O. had taken place in 1882, Freud only recalled this scene many years later.[5] By then, he had come to understand that such love was not directed towards the physician as a person but was evoked by the therapist's role. Transference love is impersonal. It relates to the specific analytic situation in which it may serve a resistive purpose – that is, the patient's unwillingness to know or to change. When patients felt drawn to Freud, he claimed to be modest enough not to attribute this to any irresistible personal charm.[6] The erotic feelings, in his view, were provoked by the analytic setting, which is characterised by a healing and helpful figure who listens and is presumed to know what ails the patient – both literally and metaphorically.

This is the Lacanian *sujet-supposé-savoir*: the psychoanalyst who is assumed to know more about the patient – or more than the patient – and who perhaps has privileged access to the meaning of life and how to find desire within it.[7] Andrea Celenza has recently emphasised the inherent seductiveness of the psychoanalytic setting: the patient's potential to fall in love is 'structured into the setting. This fact is definitional and must be accepted as a given.'[8] The analyst invariably appears as a steadfast, caring, empathic, understanding, and robust figure: ideal conditions which naturally invite the patient's desire.

DOI: 10.4324/9781003728764-19

Transference

In a paper devoted entirely to transference love, Freud argued that feelings of infatuation are merely transferred onto the analyst, as the patient unconsciously recognises earlier love figures within the analyst. More broadly, transference involves the repetition of infantile prototypes with an overwhelming sense of immediacy and actuality.[9] According to psychoanalyst and infant researcher Daniel Stern, the relationship between our infantile love life and the here-and-now of transference love shows a striking structural similarity.[10]

That Freud was always able to resist the doting and admiring love of his patients is undoubtedly due, not least, to his rigorous scientific attitude. For him, psychoanalytic treatment is fundamentally rooted in truthfulness. It is this foundation, he argued, that gives the method its educative effect and ethical value.[11] Transference love is provoked by the analytic setting, fuelled by resistance, and significantly lacking in reality testing. According to Freud, it is indifferent to consequences and even more blind than we are willing to admit to 'normal' love. When a patient falls in love with their analyst during the psychoanalytic process, everything changes. The prohibition dissolves, and the affect triumphs. Freud likens this new situation to the sudden sounding of a fire alarm during a theatrical performance.[12] He also compares this erotic coup to throwing a sausage onto a greyhound track.[13] In a famous analogy, he points out that the psychoanalyst, like a chemist, sometimes works with extremely explosive materials and must proceed with care and conscientiousness. But has chemistry ever been banned because it deals with substances that might explode?

The analyst must therefore take a firm hold of the transference. They may not respond to the patient's affection but should treat the situation as unreal and interpret it in terms of its virtuality.[14] This means tracing it back to its unconscious origin in the patient's personal history, and bringing into consciousness that which lies buried deep in the erotic life, so that the patient can once more take control of the wheel. In a later text, Freud introduces the concept of transference neurosis.[15] Within the therapeutic relationship, a kind of artificial illness emerges, in which the patient's entire pathology is enacted live on stage, unfolding within the analytic encounter. It becomes available, in every moment, for dissection. After all, problems cannot be analysed in a deeply experiential way unless they are actually occurring. The compulsion to repeat is, as it were, granted free passage to manifest within the therapeutic relationship, where – under the principle that to analyse is to suffer less or to renounce – it can be understood and worked through.[16] Former president of the *International Psychoanalytical Association*, Horacio Etchegoyen, once defined psychoanalysis in a single sentence: 'Psychoanalysis is a method that recognises the past in the present and distinguishes it by means of interpretation.'[17]

The Gift

As a therapist (or, equally, as a parent, teacher, doctor, or professor), one may be offered love and adoration by desirable people on a silver platter. Or, as with Meret Oppenheim's fur-covered teacup: a ready-made, reportedly intended as a symbol of cunnilingus. Some would-be psychoanalysts in the early days were thoroughly destabilised by such temptations. Alongside Joseph Breuer, one might mention Freud's former crown prince Carl Gustav Jung and Otto Gross – both of whom Freud would later distance himself from, though for different reasons.

In his writing on the subject, Freud did not differentiate between two distinct states in which transference love might appear: one in which feelings are acted out directly or motorically, and another in which they undergo the same displacements and disguises as, for instance, in our dream life. Moreover, is a merely verbal expression like 'I love you' a psychic act or a performative one? Phrases such as 'I declare these Games open' or 'I baptise you in the name of…' are examples of acts that can only be performed through words.[18]

Contemporary authors such as Marc Hebbrecht distinguish between eroticised transference, transference love, and loving transference.[19] These reflect descending gradations of intensity, each with a relatively less disruptive – and potentially even beneficial – effect on the analytic process. Eroticised transference may assume a delirious form, characterised by sudden and intense infatuation. When the analyst responds appropriately (that is, by firmly maintaining professional boundaries), this may provoke primitive aggression in the patient. The transference then takes on psychotic proportions: it loses its 'as if' character and becomes dominated by an all-or-nothing dynamic. A well-known example is Anaïs Nin, who (after a history of incest with her father) seduced both of her psychoanalysts and, later, in her own 'analytic' practice, engaged sexually with multiple patients.[20]

In the milder form of transference love, the patient falls in love precisely because the love object is forbidden or unavailable, and thus cannot (or must not) return the feelings. Here, the 'as if' quality is preserved, and more classically neurotic and Oedipal themes predominate. Love becomes a battleground involving third parties, or the 'beloved' analyst appears, for various reasons, to be the one to blame. Loving transference, finally, marks the conclusion of a successful course of therapy. Mutual engagement, gratitude, and respect may foster warm rapport even after the therapeutic relationship has ended.

Transference Today

In general, the analyst's foundational stance today differs substantially from Freud's. Freud developed the concept of *Nachträglichkeit* (deferred action), which implies a complex, non-linear conception of time. Later events or experiences may shed new light on earlier ones, revealing fresh – particularly emotional – layers of meaning. Still, many psychoanalysts applied a kind of 'woolly mammoth' model, in which early experiences are presumed to lie frozen in time, perfectly preserved beneath the Arctic ice.[21] Today, concepts such as neutrality and abstinence are often supplemented by what is termed freely floating responsiveness. This involves the analyst taking into account their own (countertransference) feelings to better understand what is happening within the patient and in the analytic relationship.[22]

Between the two partners in the psychoanalytic dyad, a kind of shared third emerges[23] – a field of (meaning-)production that is the result of mutual co-creation.[24] This shift in analytic practice draws inspiration from a range of post-Freudian authors, but perhaps most significantly from infant research.[25] Through microanalysis of video and audio recordings of mother–infant interaction, measured at the microsecond level, we can observe the communicative components that also play a vital role in the therapeutic relationship.[26] Fully integrating these findings would go beyond the scope of this chapter and warrant a book-length treatment.[27]

In any case, psychotherapy remains, to this day, an extremely emotional and intimate undertaking. Needs and temptations can be so powerful that even the strongest professional roles and boundaries are severely tested. Rather than responding emotionally to such intense feelings, Freud unmasked them for what they truly were: intense (often erotic) childhood feelings unconsciously transferred onto the person of the therapist. In doing so, he discovered that the past can enter the psychoanalytic setting in two radically different ways. The first is in the form of memory, as anecdote: a narrative fragment that may surface from the mists of the past. The second is as a living experience in the here-and-now, in which the past repeats itself both within and outside the therapeutic relationship. This discovery remains the cornerstone of psychoanalytic therapies today, all of which seek to analyse transference and transference love as forms of resistance to awareness, and to interpret them accordingly.

Speak, Memory!

Recent developments in neurobiology confirm Freud's insights from the consulting room. Researchers now speak of two fundamentally different and neuroanatomically distinct memory systems.[28] There is the explicit, narrative, autobiographical memory system – responsible for what can be recalled, as well as for what may be repressed, for example due to shame, guilt, or fear. This system can be accessed by analysing the patient's free associations. As is well known, free association is the fundamental rule of psychoanalysis: the patient is encouraged to say whatever comes to mind, without censorship.

On the other hand, there is the implicit or procedural memory system. This system manifests as repetition. It appears in action (walking, speaking, reading, cycling) and in interaction (contact, attachment and separation, play and pleasure, consolation and mourning). In therapy, this may be interpreted as transference. The relationships and interactions formed with the early significant Other(s) are repeated and projected onto later situations and people. I emphasise: what we constructed of the early Other, because the image we formed of them is always – inevitably – coloured or distorted by fear, desire, fantasy, and so forth.

Transference love is compelling evidence that love is an artefact. For every love, in reverse, is a form of transference love. According to Freud, to find a love object is to rediscover it.[29] As Saint-Just put it: 'One always returns to one's first loves.' Jacques Lacan differs from Freud on this point and adopts a more philosophical approach. He inverts a well-known phrase by David Lynch, adding a 'w': do not look at the doughnut, but at the (w)hole.[30] For Lacan, it is not merely about the object itself, but about the lost and impossible Thing behind or within the object that seems to be rediscovered. It is this unattainable aim, he argues, that determines the subject's orientation towards the (love) object. For as such, the original love object is naturally and by definition unfindable and unreachable. It exists, so to speak, only as some aria: *La Donna Che Non Si Trova*.[31] Lacan elaborates these ideas in an entire seminar year devoted to transference and Plato's *Symposium*.[32]

Analysts (like Socrates, the protagonist of Plato's dialogue) pose many questions to which the patient has little or no answer. In doing so, they magnify the patient's sense of lack, even as the patient begins to believe that the analyst 'knows' precisely because the analyst asks such apt questions. The patient becomes a lover of the analyst, imagining that something in the analyst responds to what is lacking in themselves. They perceive a 'something' in the analyst. This is the *agalma* or *object petit a*: the treasure that (the otherwise hideous) Socrates, according to the beautiful Alcibiades, secretly holds within. This psychodynamic underpins Socrates' maieutic, or midwifery, method, on which psychoanalysis is based: truths are drawn from the patient. These truths can be found only in the patient's unconscious and must be deciphered and translated by someone who may not know the content but who understands the language of the unconscious.

Who Knows?

Ironically, the patient believes they know themselves well, whereas the analyst knows they know very little. In the analytic situation, knowledge flows not from the analyst to the patient, but from the analyst's lack of knowledge to the patient. Referring to Lacan's definition of love as 'to give what one does not have,' this is the analyst's way of giving. Because analysts thus encourage patients to explore desires that often conflict with social norms, they may also share in Socrates' fate: banishment to the margins.

According to Lacan, the patient is placed in the position of the beloved. By speaking, he seeks to be loved, and the therapist treats him or her as someone who matters, listening in a way he or she has perhaps never been listened to before. The therapist's love must not burst into flame but smoulder, like a damp log on the hearth.[33] He occupies a unique position: he must love without wishing to be loved in return. He does not assume the position of the beloved but that of the lover, provoking the patient to know (Socrates compares himself to a gadfly). He is merely a shareholder in the knowledge inscribed in the patient's unconscious.

In him, too (as in Socrates), there appears to reside a dazzling and fascinating 'something' that Lacan calls object petit a, an element that imaginatively veils the Thing. The patient's transference-love is the motor of the analytic work, yet the analyst is not its object. Rather, he is the object-cause of desire (Lacan's *objet petit a*), the element that sets desire in motion, and he must strive for 'discourse in the stead of intercourse': verbal rather than sexual relations.[34] He loves the patient's soul (the unconscious) and is glad to see him or her arrive, but not to reach completion with or through the patient.

The therapist is not free of any (including erotic) feelings for the patient, yet he does not ventilate them, for his concern lies elsewhere. In his non-desire to cure, he distances himself from excessive therapeutic ambition or the fury to heal (the so-called *furor sanandi*). What he seeks is simply to encounter the patient's unconscious in its innumerable manifestations. During his own formation as a psychoanalyst, a necessary transformation must have occurred in the economy of his desire. The analyst may love or hate as much as anyone else, yet a different relation between love, desire, and drive has been established in him, resulting in a kind of *tough love*.[35] In his interventions, he mainly marks the patient's own expressions (those that repeat themselves in one way or another) and speaks as little as possible in his own name. He does not seek to be loved, but merely to help bring the patient's unconscious into speech.[36]

Genuine

The patient's transference love for the therapist is a genuine form of love, and the feelings involved are entirely authentic. Yet this love is subject to specific conditions. It lends itself particularly well to analysis (and to the analysis of resistance) because it is even more strictly determined by the past than romantic love. It is a pure unconscious creation of the person involved. This naturally raises questions about the status of reality versus illusion: what is real, and what is virtual? Transference, then, functions as an intermediate zone between illness and real life, through which the transformation from one to the other can be realised in therapy.[37]

Psychoanalysis is especially interested in love for two reasons. Firstly, disturbances in the capacity to love are among the most common motives for seeking analytic treatment. But above all, transference love (so long as it remains unreciprocated) is the driving force of the psychoanalytic process itself. The oft-repeated critique of the lengthy duration of analysis and its supposed induction of dependency is therefore misguided. Problems are not caused by the analysis, but uncovered by it. Gradually, transference and transference love are worked through and resolved. For within analysis, they receive special treatment. Alongside dreams, they form the royal road (the *via regia*) to knowledge of the unconscious and of repetition.

The psychoanalytic relationship is a unique form of love, precisely because amorous exaltation is sublimated into a source of knowledge through abstention. Unlike other impossible or forbidden loves, transference love is not rejected. On the contrary, it restores to the person concerned their dignity and freedom – perhaps more so than ever before. Transference allows us to free ourselves from repetition and opens up alternative possibilities. It enables us to discover, among other things, new and different ways of loving and of experiencing pleasure.

Notes

1 Freud, S. (1912). *Adviezen voor de arts bij de psychoanalytische behandeling* (pp. 87–99). K.B.4. Sigmund Freud Nederlandse Editie. Amsterdam/Meppel: Boom.
2 Breuer, J., & Freud, S. (1895). *Studies over hysterie*. K.B.5. Sigmund Freud Nederlandse Editie. Amsterdam/Meppel: Boom.
3 Sulloway, F. (1979). *Freud: Biologist of the mind* (p. 77). New York: Basic Books.
4 Jones, E. (1953). *The life and work of Sigmund Freud* (pp. 222–226). London: Hogarth.
5 Sulloway, F. (1979). *Freud: Biologist of the mind* (p. 80). New York: Basic Books.
6 Freud, S. (1916/1917). Introductory lectures on psycho-analysis. In *Standard edition* (Vols. 15–16, p. 450). London: Hogarth Press.
7 Lacan, J. (2024). *Le Séminaire. Livre XV. L'Acte psychanalytique*. Texte établi par J. A. Miller. Paris: Seuil.
8 Celenza, A. (2007). Analytic love and power: Responsiveness and responsibility. *Psychoanalytic Inquiry*, *27*, 298.
9 Laplanche, J., & Pontalis, J. B. (1967). *Vocabulaire de la psychanalyse*. Paris: PUF.
10 Stern, D. (1993/2018). Acting versus remembering in transference love and infantile love. In E. Person, A. Hagelin, & P. Fonagy (Eds.), *On Freud's 'Observations on transference-love'*. London/New York: Routledge.
11 Freud, S. (1916/1917). Introductory lectures on psycho-analysis. In *Standard edition* (Vols. 15–16, p. 434) en Freud, S. (1933). New introductory lectures on psychoanalysis. In *Standard edition* (Vol. 20, p. 182). London: Hogarth Press.
12 Freud, S. (1915). Verdere adviezen over de psychoanalytische techniek (III). Opmerkingen over overdrachtsliefde. In *Freud werken* (pp. 434–4447). Amsterdam: Boom.
13 Freud, S. (1915). Verdere adviezen over de psychoanalytische techniek (III). Opmerkingen over overdrachtsliefde. In *Freud werken* (pp. 434–4447). Amsterdam: Boom.
14 Freud, S. (1900). The interpretation of dreams. In *Freud standard edition* (Vols. 4–5, p. 611): 'everything that can be an object of our internal perception is virtual, like the image produced in a telescope by the passage of lightrays'. London: Hogarth Press
15 Freud, S. (1914). *Herinneren, herhalen en doorwerken*. K.B.4. Sigmund Freud Nederlandse Editie. Amsterdam/Meppel: Boom.
16 Freud, S. (1914). *Herinneren, herhalen en doorwerken*. K.B.4. Sigmund Freud Nederlandse Editie. Amsterdam/Meppel: Boom.
17 Etchegoyen, R. H. (1999). *The fundamentals of psychoanalytic technique* (p. 112). London/New York: Karnac.
18 Searle, J. R. (1969). *Speech acts: An essay in the philosophy of language*. New York: Cambridge University Press.
19 Hebbrecht, M. (2006). In de ban van overdrachtsliefde. *Tijdschrift voor Psychoanalyse 4*, 301–315.
20 Bair, D. (1996). *Anaïs Nin – Biografie*. Baarn: Anthos.
21 Wachtel, P. L. (2003). The surface and depths: The metaphor of depth in psychoanalysis and the ways it can mislead. *Contemporary Psychoanalysis*, *39*(1), 22.
22 Sandler, J. (1976). Countertransference and role-responsiveness. *International Review of Psycho-Analysis*, *3*(1), 43–47.
23 Ogden, T. H. (2004). The analytic third: Implications for psychoanalytic theory and technique. *The Psychoanalytic Quarterly*, *73*(1), 167–195.
24 Civitarese, G. (2021). Intersubjectivity and analytic field theory. *Journal of the American Psychoanalytic Association*, *69*(5), 853–893.
25 Harrison, A. M., & Beebe, B. (2018). Rhythms of dialogue in infant research and child analysis: Implicit and explicit forms of therapeutic action. *Psychoanalytic Psychology*, *35*(4), 367.

26 Zhang, W., Pan, Q., & Guo, B. The significance of infant research for psychoanalysis. *Humanities and Social Sciences Communications (Nature)*, *9*, 194.
27 Kinet, M. (2024). *Psychoanalytic principles in psychiatric practice. A remedy by truth.* London/New York: Routledge.
28 Kinet, M. (2023). *The spirit of the drive in neuropsychoanalysis*. London/New York: Routledge.
29 Freud, S. (1905). *Drie verhandelingen over de theorie van de seksualiteit* (pp. 49–177). K.B.1. Sigmund Freud Nederlandse Editie. Amsterdam/Meppel: Boom.
30 Rodley, C. (1997). *Lynch on Lynch. Interviews*. London: Faber.
31 Carotenuto, A. (1982/1992). *La donna che non si trova* (Nuova ed.). Milano: Bompiani.
32 Lacan, J. (1960–1961/1991). *Le Séminaire. Livre VIII. Le transfert*. Texte établi par J. A. Miller. Paris: Du Seuil.
33 Allouch, J. (2009). *L'amour Lacan*. Paris: Epel.
34 Fink, B. (2015). *Lacan on love: An exploration of Lacan's seminar VIII, transference*. New York: Polity.
35 The Italian psychoanalyst Piera Aulagnier famously introduced the concept of 'the violence of interpretation': the psychical action by which one imposes on another's psyche a choice, a thought or an action that is motivated by the desire of the person who imposes it, but which is based on an object that responds for the other to the category of the necessary. Aulagnier, P. (2001). *The violence of interpretation* (p. 13). London/New York: Routledge.
36 Lacan, J. (1960–1961/1991). *Le Séminaire. Livre VIII. Le transfert*. Texte établi par J. A. Miller. Paris: Du Seuil.
37 Eickhoff, F. W. (1987). A short annotation to Sigmund Freud's 'Observations on transference-love'. *The International Journal of Psycho-Analysis*, *14*, 103–109.

18

A Loving Place

Setting the Stage

The psychoanalytic setting may well be Freud's most important technical contribution. It creates a space for thinking thoughts that have not yet been thought, for speaking words that have never (quite) been spoken before, and for expressing feelings that have never been experienced in this way.[1] Psychoanalysis is thus not only a theory, a clinical practice, and a method of inquiry into the human mind. It also realises a very particular kind of relationship[2] – one that Freud himself described as 'unmatched in real life.'[3]

Today, this therapeutic relationship is regarded as the vehicle and matrix of the analytic process. Sooner or later, our history – that is, the unconscious – steps live onto the stage of the analytic encounter, allowing it to be recognised and worked through.[4] A good therapeutic relationship is now also seen as a paradigmatic, non-specific factor. It has demonstrable efficacy regardless of the theoretical model employed.[5] Moreover, it is considered a necessary condition for therapeutic effectiveness. It is not sufficient: even in the most trusting of relationships, there may be little lasting change in unconscious psychodynamics, psychogenesis, or classically conflict-based neuroses unless transference reactions or distortions – and the interplay of inner forces – are recognised, verbalised, and interpreted as such.

For Erich Fromm, psychoanalytic therapy is above all aimed at restoring the patient's capacity to love.[6] A classic work on psychoanalytic technique by Karl Menninger explicitly states that the goal of a successful analysis is for the patient to learn how to live: 'that is, to love and to be loved.'[7] As early as 1906, in a letter to then-crown prince Carl Gustav Jung, Freud referred to psychoanalysis as '*Eigentlich eine Heilung durch Liebe.*'[8] An almost identical phrase appears in a 1909 letter to Max Eitingon: 'the secret of therapy is to cure through love.'[9] In *Civilisation and Its Discontents*, Freud concludes that the best path for human life is one that places love at the centre and finds fulfilment in loving and being loved.[10] Contemporary happiness research confirms this: friendships, family ties, and romantic relationships are among the strongest predictors of well-being.[11]

DOI: 10.4324/9781003728764-20

The Love Cure

It was Sandor Ferenczi who, more than anyone after Freud, emphasised the central role of love in the psychoanalytic cure.[12] According to Ferenczi, an all-conquering love is a necessary condition for successful therapy. 'No analysis can succeed if we do not succeed in really loving the patient.'[13] In a modest way, I identify with Ferenczi in several respects. Like him, I began as a (psychiatric) hospital physician working with some of the 'sickest' and most challenging (often socioeconomically disadvantaged) patients. These were a very different type of patient from the predominantly neurotic Viennese bourgeoisie Freud treated – clients who, per session, paid the equivalent of a working man's weekly wage.[14] Emotional neglect, abuse, and maltreatment were rampant in Ferenczi's clinical practice. Many theoretical and technical disagreements among even the most famous psychoanalysts can be traced to the distinct patient populations and challenges they encountered.

For my part, I consider the analytic couch and a rigid distance from the analyst ill-advised in such cases. Everyone ought to watch Edward Tronick's *YouTube* videos of the *Still Face* experiment to understand what a blank face does to (the baby in) us.[15] The technique must remain sufficiently elastic and, where necessary, draw on methods used by psychoanalytic play therapists.[16] Like children, many of these patients are not yet sufficiently able to express themselves solely through language.

According to legend, Ferenczi even would have cured a sick horse.[17] The therapeutic zeal for which he is sometimes criticised seems to me a compliment: I have never quite understood what's supposedly so wrong with a bit of 'curative rage' (*furor sanandi*) – the excesses of which, ironically, were precisely what Michael Balint would later critique.[18] This doesn't imply any feeling of omnipotence on the part of the therapist. After all, don't parents – and by extension, therapists – sometimes need to fight for their child's (or patient's) life? A newborn will not survive unless the parents mobilise everything they have on their behalf. Even being merely 'unwanted' can be (literally or figuratively) deadly to a child.[19] I will return to this.

The Usual Suspect

The therapeutic relationship is often described as isomorphic with the parent–child relationship. While they differ in many respects, they share analogous dynamics regarding rights and responsibilities, as well as the framework within which interaction can or may occur. The approach of psychoanalysts such as Ferenczi, Michael Balint, or Donald Winnicott has sometimes been (somewhat dismissively) described as more parental than psychoanalytic. Yet one need only read Winnicott's *Holding and Interpretation* to realise – through its detailed case material – that their analyses by no means reduced the patient to the role of a son or daughter, nor the analyst to that of a benevolent parent.[20] That said, most contemporary analysts now attribute significant therapeutic efficacy to what Ferenczi first introduced as the introjection of a healing experience within the therapeutic relationship.[21]

As a psychiatrist, often confronted with patients who neither request nor imagine psychotherapy (let alone psychoanalysis), I can wholeheartedly confirm this. An active psychotherapist who offers timely and thoughtful interpretation, who mentalises, or who constructs a working model of the patient's internal world or history, can provide an immensely helpful, even life-saving, intervention. Without this sort of preparatory labour, strictly interpretative, 'pure' analytic work often cannot begin at all. Ferenczi had already understood this a century ago.[22]

In part due to various (often sensationalised) erotic entanglements between patient and therapist, love has acquired a somewhat suspicious (if not downright tainted) connotation within psychoanalysis. Yet love, in general, resists definition, and this is equally true for its psychoanalytic variant. It may resemble parental love, fraternal love, neighbourly love, friendship, and so on – but it is 'not simply or actually any of those… It is a thing unto itself.'[23]

Therapeutic Love

According to infant researcher and psychoanalyst Daniel Stern, it is characterised by the analyst's sustained effort to ensure that all their feelings (and the behaviours that flow from them) are in the patient's best interests and conducive to the patient's psychic growth.[24] He even suggests that, under such conditions, genuine and spontaneous expressions of love on the part of the analyst can be extremely 'powerful and transformative.'[25]

The therapist's role is often compared to Donald Winnicott's idea of 'good-enough mothering.'[26] I believe this is inaccurate. The analyst's deep commitment to the patient's psyche is more akin to Winnicott's notion of 'primary maternal preoccupation.'[27] Most parents experience heightened sensitivity towards their baby during this period – a biological and psychosocial preparedness. An analogue in psychoanalysis is Lacan's so-called 'desire of the analyst,' nourished by one's own analysis and by solid theoretical and clinical training. This combination creates a kind of 'second self' that is consistently benevolent and loving.

Roy Schafer argues that, at their best, analysts are not quite the same people in sessions as they are in their everyday social lives or personal relationships. During the session, they are often 'better' human beings, in the sense that they empathise more and in a more accepting and effective manner. He concludes (in my own translation): 'On this basis, a particular kind of empathic intimacy, strength, appreciation, and love can develop in the relationship with the analysand – and it would be a mistake to equate this with disruptive countertransference.'[28] Otto Kernberg observes that, outside clinical situations, analysts are simply human[29]: they become defensive when criticised, they sometimes avoid intimacy, and they may become easily irritated. And yet, within the psychoanalytic setting, they can readily attain a level of empathy that is rare in ordinary life. He adds: perhaps this has something to do with the 'genius of the psychoanalytic situation' – as a method for finding some measure of happiness and for alleviating suffering?[30]

This also concerns the so-called 'special moments' in psychotherapy. They can be prepared for or facilitated, but not planned. These often involve work at deeper layers of the psyche, where the patient is released from unspoken, disruptive contents (akin to the maieutic or midwifery method of Socrates or the psychoanalyst). This occurs because the analyst can fruitfully use their own subjectivity[31] (partly shaped by countertransference) to receive, contain, and transform such contents before offering them back. This inner work involves disturbing feelings or thoughts in the analyst, which help them to weigh, cradle, and ultimately return the material in a modified form.[32]

This psychic crib 'functions' according to Bion's container-contained model, and enables so-called 'moments of meeting' in which an unbearable experience can be narratively co-constructed by the analytic couple. Patient and therapist may truly feel 'in sync' at such moments.[33] Independent of insight, these experiences deepen and intensify the therapeutic relationship.[34] They can therefore play a significant role in the transformation that therapy seeks to achieve.

The Basic Fault

Finally, I wish to turn to the problem of the *basic fault* as described by Michael Balint.[35] For such patients, the therapeutic relationship may be the first – and perhaps only – place where they can experience what love truly entails. I quote from an email written by Tania, who for many years has been one of my most vulnerable 'worry children' and immediately comes to mind in this context:

> In nearly 44 years, I haven't managed to find anyone who truly cares about me (except professionals). Not even my parents. No one in the outside world. Absolutely no one! I am a burden. That's what I mean to people: a deep sigh. I asked my sister to look for garden fertiliser at *Aldi* when she went shopping in her area. It's only a one-minute drive. I told her there was none left near me. Even that is too much for her. I no longer know what or whom I'm living for. No one loves me. And you can't force it. I've done everything I could to be loved… I'm like a skunk… No one loves me. What happens when you're gone?

Tania has felt unseen and unloved her entire life: misunderstood, orphaned, a fifth wheel, a *quantité négligeable*. She is the youngest of three daughters. The two eldest were wanted and, through their appearance and school performance, met their parents' expectations – self-employed and hardworking, and therefore often absent. They are now seemingly doing well in psychosocial and societal terms. Tania, by contrast, remembers watching her own family through her bedroom window, and also looking through other people's windows in search of cosy, domestic scenes. As a teenager, she literally taped SOS messages behind the wallpaper. She often escaped into fairy tales and fantasy films. In particular, she identified with

Rémi from Hector Malot's novel *Sans Famille.*[36] She worked hard at home and at school but was repeatedly bullied and excluded.

She lost her mother to cancer at a young age, and due to her caring role, she witnessed the suffering and deterioration from up close. Since adolescence, she has been in continuous psychotherapy and was institutionalised in a youth psychiatric setting. With encouragement and support, she studied nursing and worked for several years 'like a Duracell bunny.' She poured herself into caring for patients and colleagues, and, while working in an oncology ward, witnessed what she described as many 'inhuman' situations. Her father (with whom she at least shared moments of laughter) died a few years ago, leaving her literally and emotionally orphaned. Following major conflicts with her sisters over inheritance, and a serious suicide attempt, she underwent a prolonged clinical psychotherapeutic treatment during which she remained deeply separation-anxious and regressed, clinging to the mother-figure embodied by the environment and its caregivers. While her capacity for insight and mentalisation grew significantly, there was also considerable ego regression, and many of her (literal and figurative) 'muscles' atrophied within the protective hospital environment. Alongside psychotherapy, rehabilitation is now essential.

Subtle

In other patients, the issue is less pronounced because they function more effectively in social or professional contexts. Much psychological suffering remains both invisible and misunderstood. I think of Rita, a woman in her late forties who has been in weekly therapy for several years. She is the younger of two children. Her mother once considered an abortion. While extremely caring in practical and material ways, her mother appears chronically misattuned and unaware of what her daughter truly needs or enjoys. Her brother, two years older, reportedly treated her harshly and with persistent hostility.

At one point, Rita likened herself to the princess in *The Princess and the Pea*, but now she often breaks into tears, saying the pea has become 'a bed of nails.' She feels unwanted and rejected everywhere she goes, never greeted with a smile or a 'good morning,' never welcomed – not even, as she says, 'from the very beginning.'

Then there is Jenny. She initially presented as a clever, independent, and free-spirited young woman with unexplained anxiety and depression that seemed to arise 'out of nowhere.' After nearly 20 years of continuous psychotherapy (ranging from 24-hour residential care to outpatient therapy), it became vividly clear that she, like Snow White, had a narcissistic mother who denied her daughter everything – even going so far as to take away her few belongings and gifts. To make matters worse, Jenny is infertile due to a combination of parental negligence and repeated dismissals of her endometriosis symptoms by various (in her view, narcissistic) gynaecologists. Eventually, she had to undergo surgical removal of her uterus and ovaries – a procedure historically referred to as 'castration.' She carries with her a sometimes 'unbearable void' in her heart (and abdomen), compounded by the irretrievable loss of any hope for motherhood or a warm, loving family of her own.

What About the Basics?

The *basic fault* is a central concept in the work of Hungarian-British psychoanalyst Michael Balint. It refers to a profound disruption in the early mother–child relationship, typically occurring in the first months of life, before personality formation. From Balint's perspective, it is a fundamental absence or deficiency that arises when the primary need for a safe, responsive, and emotionally nurturing relationship with a caregiver is not adequately met. It does not result in an intrapsychic conflict (as in classical Freudian theory), but in a psychic void – a kind of existential rupture in the self.

It concerns a pre-Oedipal issue rooted in developmental failure. It gives rise to feelings of emptiness, anxiety, emotional dependence, and – not least – a longing for regression. I sometimes allude to the words of the Dutch poet Gerrit Achterberg: '*I wish I were a calf that rests beside its mother.*'[37] In such cases, the focus shifts away from interpretation and towards the provision (and sustained offering) of a holding environment. Regression is not seen as resistance or flight, but rather as a possible – if not the only –path towards healing. What matters most is the therapist's ability to continue bearing the regression, rather than rejecting or needlessly commenting on the patient's persistent 'sighing' (as in Tania's case).

'There seems to be a fault, a basic fault in the structure of the personality, a fault that cannot be repaired by the usual means of interpretation or insight.'[38] And again: 'Regression to the basic fault is not an obstacle to therapy but potentially the therapy itself.'[39]

This is a matter of *primary object love*: an early and foundational form of love that arises in the first moments of the child's life – typically with the mother or another primary caregiver. This love is not sexual but expresses a deep longing for fusion, unity, and safety. It is a form of love in which the child does not yet experience itself as separate from the other. It is primarily nonverbal, bodily, and affective. It is about feeling, sensing, being held – about simply being allowed to exist in the presence of the other, without the necessity of *doing* anything.[40]

The absence of such love may lie at the heart of a patient's suffering, but it is even more often an aspect or component of broader experiences of neglect, abuse, or psychological trauma. Balint viewed this form of love as legitimate and not necessarily pathological – provided the therapist is capable of receiving and holding the regressive love without being overwhelmed by it. It lies at the core of what is sometimes called the therapy of *presence* (as opposed to *intervention*).[41] In our highly technical times, this kind of presence risks becoming increasingly rare...

Notes

1 Künstlicher, R. (1996). The function of the frame. *Scandinavian Psychoanalytic Review, 19*, 164.
2 Steingart, I. (1995). *A thing apart: Love and reality in the therapeutic relationship* (pp. 108–109). Northvale: Jason Aronson.
3 Freud, S. (1915). Observations on transference-love (Further recommendations on the technique of psycho-analysis III). In *Freud standard edition* (Vol. 12, p. 166). London: Hogarth Press.
4 Kinet, M. (2024). *Psychoanalytic principles in psychiatric practice. A remedy by truth.* London/New York: Routledge.
5 Hubble, M. A., Duncan, B. L., & Miller, S. D. (1999). *The heart and soul of change: What works in therapy.* New York: American Psychological Association.
6 Fromm, E. (1950). *Psychoanalysis and religion* (p. 87). New Haven: Yale University Press.
7 Menninger, K. (1958). *Theory of psychoanalytic technique* (pp. 178–179). New York: Basic Books.
8 Freud, S. (1906/1974). Letter from Sigmund Freud to C. G. Jung, December 6, 1906. In W. McGuire (Ed.), *The Freud/Jung letters: The correspondence between Sigmund Freud and C. G. Jung* (pp. 11–13). Princeton: Princeton University Press.
9 Falzeder, E. (1994). My grand patient, my chief tormentor: A hitherto unnoticed case of Freud's and the consequences. *Psychoanalytic Quarterly, 63*, 310.
10 Freud, S. (1930). Civilization and its discontents. In *Freud standard edition* (Vol. 21, pp. 80–81). London: Hogarth Press.
11 Waldinger, R. J., & Schulz, M. S. (2023). *The good life: Lessons from the world's longest scientific study of happiness.* New York: Simon & Schuster.
12 De Vleminck, J. (2018). Ohne Sympathie keine Heilung: Sándor Ferenczi en de analytische techniek. *Tijdschrift voor Psychoanalyse, 24*(2), 127–129.
13 Ferenczi, S. (1932/1988). *The clinical diary of Sandor Ferenczi* (pp. 129–130). Cambridge: Harvard University Press.
14 Onfray, M. (2010). *Le crépuscule d'une idole. L'affabulation freudienne.* Paris: Grasset.
15 Tronick, E. (2007). *The neurobehavioral and social-emotional development of infants and children.* London/New York: Norton. https://youtu.be/f1Jw0-LExyc
16 Kinet, M. (2024). *Psychoanalytic principles in psychiatric practice. A remedy by truth.* London/New York: Routledge.
17 Ferenczi, S. (1913/1955). Taming of a wild horse. In *Final contributions to the problems and methods of psycho-analysis* (pp. 336–340). London: Hogarth.
18 Balint, M. (1964). *The doctor, his patient and the illness.* London: Pitman Medical.
19 Ferenczi, S. (1929/1955). The unwelcome child and his death instinct. In *Final contributions to the problems and methods of psycho-analysis* (pp. 102–107). London: Hogarth.
20 Winnicott, D. W. (1986). *Holding and interpretation: Fragment of an analysis.* London: Karnac Books, 1989.
21 Ferenczi, S. (1909/1970). Introjektion und Übertragung. In *Schriften zur Psychoanalyse* (pp. 12–47). Frankfurt am Main: Fischer Verlag.
22 Kinet, M. (2023). Enkele voorlaatste woorden. Tussen ça voir en faire ainsi. In M. Hebbrecht & C. Franckx (Red.), *Het kinderlijk trauma. Verloren tussen tederheid en passie* (pp. 295–306). Antwerpen/'s Hertogenbosch: Gompel&Svacina.
23 Shaw, D. (2003). On the therapeutic action of analytic love. *Contemporary Psychoanalysis, 39*, 268.
24 Stern, S. (2011). The therapeutic action of analytic love: Commentary on Joye Weisel-Barth's "Katherine: A long, hard case". *International Journal of Psycho-Analysis, 6*, 489–504.

25 Stern, S. (2011). The therapeutic action of analytic love: Commentary on Joye Weisel-Barth's "Katherine: A long, hard case". *International Journal of Psycho-Analysis, 6*, 497.

26 Winnicott, D. W. (1965). *The maturational processes and the facilitating environment: Studies in the theory of emotional development.* London: Hogarth Press.

27 Lev, G. (2023). Conditions for love: The psychoanalytic situation and the analyst's emotions. *International Forum of Psychoanalysis, 32*(2), 120.

28 Schafer, R. (1983). *The analytic attitude* (p. 291). New York: Basic Books.

29 Kernberg, O. F. (1994). Love in the analytic setting. *Journal of the American Psychoanalytic Association, 42*, 1147.

30 Bienvenu, J. (2003). Healing through the search for truth. *Canadian Journal of Psychoanalysis, 11*, 408.

31 Ginnieri-Coccossis, M., & Vaslamatzis, G. (2014). Truths, reveries, internal moments of meeting: Reflections on the dialectics of the analytic relationship. *International Forum of Psychoanalysis, 23*, 171–82.

32 Gabbard, G. O., & Ogden, T. H. (2009). On becoming a psychoanalyst. *International Journal of Psychoanalysis, 9*, 311–327.

33 Békés, V., & Hoffman, L. (2021). The "something" more than working alliance: Authentic relational moments. *Journal of the American Psychoanalytic Association, 68*, 1051–1064.

34 The Boston Change Process Study Group. (2010). *Change in psychotherapy. A unifying paradigm.* New York: Norton.

35 Balint, M. (1968). *The basic fault: Therapeutic aspects of regression.* London: Tavistock Publications.

36 Malot, H. (1878/1999). *Alleen op de wereld* (A. Willemsen, Vert.). Amsterdam: De Arbeiderspers.

37 Achterberg, G. (1945/2008). Eiland der ziel. In *Verzamelde gedichten* (S. Vestdijk & G. Kamphuis, Red.). Amsterdam: Querido.

38 Balint, M. (1968). *The basic fault: Therapeutic aspects of regression* (p. 96). London: Tavistock Publications.

39 Casement, P. (1990). *Further learning from the patient* (p. 143). London/New York: Routledge.

40 Balint, M. (1952). *Primary love and psychoanalytic technique* (p. 46). London: Hogarth Press.

41 Baart, A. (2001). *Een theorie van de presentie.* Utrecht: Lemma.

19

The Couple on the Couch?

Apology

In our small yet complex Belgium, we have five governments and three official languages: Dutch, French, and German. I belong to the Flemish/Dutch-speaking part of the country, where these three languages are systematically taught alongside English. Flanders occupies a culturally minoritised position: prestige is often granted only when one succeeds 'abroad.' The saying that no one is a prophet in their own land was probably coined here. Yet every disadvantage has its benefit. Flemings have absorbed a wide range of cultural influences, which have yielded considerable beauty in the arts and the humanities. This context explains why, in this chapter on psychoanalytic couple therapy, I draw freely from English, German, and French traditions.

In contemporary clinical practice and cultural diagnostics, there is a growing need for an integrated conceptual framework that can situate both desire and stagnation within couple relationships. Three figures offer complementary perspectives: Esther Perel, with her relational and culturally informed idea of 'erotic intelligence'; Jürg Willi, with his systemic-psychoanalytic analysis of collusion; and Jacques Lacan, with his theorisation of the symptom, the fantasy, and unconscious desire. What unites them is the conviction that love is not merely an emotional affair but a structured phenomenon, shaped by the unconscious and by the way the subject constructs itself through the Other. As will become clear, I align most closely with the latter two. This has much to do with my persistent suspicion of any Promised Land. Does *Brave New World* not teach us that every utopia inevitably implies (and simultaneously threatens to become) a dystopia?[1]

The Promised Land

Genital love, introduced in Freud's theory of psychosexual development, encompasses the integration of sexual and aggressive impulses as well as the capacity to invest libido in external and whole (as opposed to partial or narcissistic) objects. For Freud, it represents a developmental achievement linked to the resolution of the Oedipus complex and the establishment of stable object relations.[2] A similar

DOI: 10.4324/9781003728764-21

conception is found in Michael Balint, who holds that such love involves reciprocity, intimacy, and trust, and requires recognising the partner as a separate individual.[3] More recently, Otto Kernberg has endorsed and elaborated this position in his structural developmental model, emphasising the integration of self- and object representations and the capacity to tolerate ambivalence. In his view, mature love synthesises libidinal drive, object constancy, and ego maturation.[4]

Lacanian thought is often criticised for offering slogans that seem carved in stone and repeated (untouched) by disciples from Africa to America, from the Himalayas to the desert. Yet these formulations each capture Lacan's fundamental axiom: the Real (by definition) cannot be symbolised. *La femme n'existe pas. Il n'y a pas d'Autre de l'Autre.* Or, most relevant here, *Il n'y a pas de rapport sexuel.*[5] They all revolve around the idea that the Real of drive and trauma can never be fully articulated and never fully integrated. Love and desire are attempts to repair what never was. They are structurally doomed to fail – yet it is precisely in the pulse of this attempt that subjectivation takes place. I refer to Samuel Beckett: 'Ever tried. Ever failed. No matter. Try again. Fail again. Fail better.'[6] With this premise, Lacan blows apart the (psycho-)logical ideal of so-called 'mature, genital love.' Just as there is inevitably a *rencontre manquée*[7] (a missed encounter) between mother and child, so there is between lovers. To explore the consequences for psychoanalytically oriented couple therapy, I begin on a more positive note.

Perel Harbour

Esther Perel is an American psychotherapist, author, and renowned speaker on relationships, sexuality, and 'modern love.' She is frequently cited in the media, including *The New York Times*, *The Guardian*, and *The New Yorker,* perhaps because her message is optimistic.[8] She emphasises the development of erotic intelligence through which difficulties in couples might be managed.[9] She attempts to bridge the tension between safety and intimacy on the one hand and excitement or sexuality on the other. Her approach, in my view, has something of an interior-decorating quality: the unconscious and the partners' histories remain largely unaddressed. Instead, the central question becomes: through which interventions can eroticism be kept alive in long-term relationships? Desire requires distance and mystery, which inevitably runs counter to the trust and familiarity characteristic of enduring partnerships. For Perel, the central issue is often how one feels in the presence of the partner. Eroticism is first and foremost a self-experience in the presence of the other: do we feel sufficiently free, playful, and powerful in each other's company? This experiential basis, rather than the relationship itself, becomes the primary therapeutic focus.

Eroticism requires sufficient psychic space. This resonates with Lacan's idea that desire is fuelled by distance, and with the notion that the Other must remain partly enigmatic, for knowing the Other 'too well' tends to extinguish erotic fire. Perel, therefore, warns against excessive or constant proximity. There must be enough transitional space, à la Winnicott, to facilitate play, creativity, and fantasy.[10]

When this playful space collapses, the couple risks an erotically dead relationship. Her 'erotic intelligence' is not about sexual gymnastics, but about how we can continue to integrate fantasy, transgression, and play into our erotic lives. She normalises erotic role-play and appeals to the link between excitement and transgression (taboo, dominance–submission, the forbidden), where adventures can be staged in a 'safe' manner (like in an amusement park). Partners can play with power, vulnerability, or identity in ways that never surface in daylight. Since Freud, we know that infantile sexuality is polymorphous, perverse, and saturated with fantasy and symbolism. Perel emphasises that these elements must remain part of the erotic relationship.

Kleinian ideas about ambivalence and the depressive position also illuminate couples' emotional complexities.[11] When partners try to cover everything 'for the sake of peace,' they may repress aggression or fantasy, thereby flattening the erotic dynamic. Conflict and its repair, distance and reconciliation, lose their animating (and eroticising) potential. Consistent with Jean Laplanche's theory of generalised seduction, the Other must remain sufficiently enigmatic (sufficiently 'traumatic') to stimulate the sexual.[12] Erotic logic lies at the limit of the pleasure principle. For Perel, the resurgence of desire in real or fantasised affairs is often a *quest for aliveness*.[13]

The erotic vitality that accompanies such awakenings breaks the deadening effect of duty and routine, domesticity, and predictability. Erotic adventures may be dangerous and therefore transgressive. They may exceed the pleasure principle and move onto the slippery ice of Lacanian *jouissance*.[14] The couple remains alive only insofar as it preserves openness to this fantasmatic space. Desire often flares when we observe our partner from a distance, in a context where they appear independent, self-aware, and (thus) attractive to others. Rekindling desire is less about solving problems than shifting perspectives. Let me now shift to the German tradition.

Willy Nilly

Jürg Willi was a Swiss psychiatrist and psychoanalyst best known for his pioneering work on partner relationships in a systemic-psychoanalytic framework.[15] His central concept is *collusion*: an unconscious, often neurotic conspiracy between two partners, in which both adopt complementary roles allowing them to relive unresolved childhood conflicts in a kind of vicarious 'solution' through the other. Partner choice is not accidental but symptomatic, based on unconscious, fantasmatic complementarities. Under the cloak of love, each partner confirms the other's neurosis. Initially, collusion acts as cement and a magnet, but it gradually leads to stagnation or conflict.

Willi distinguishes four main forms of collusion, depending on the dominant conflict enacted in the relationship. I mention only the three clearest. In narcissistic collusion, there is the star and the admirer: one idolises, the other is idolised. Problems of low or fragile self-esteem are thus 'managed.' In oral collusion, we observe the caregiver and the cared-for revolving around early-childhood deficits. In Oedipal collusion, parent–child roles predominate not in terms of care but in terms of power, authority, or rivalry. Complementary transferences lead to stereotyped interactions and repeated conflict. In all these configurations, partners choose each other through transferential and/or projective mechanisms. The collusion can yield positive outcomes and provide emotional gratification, but more often a childhood drama is reenacted live on stage without catharsis or insight. It leads only to painful and exhausting repetition. Therapy is insight-oriented: its aim is not to determine who is right, but to recognise one's own part in the *pas-de-deux*.

Willi's approach clearly seeks deep and often confronting insight into how love, dependency, anxiety, and unconscious repetition converge within intimate space. The relationship is analysed through classical psychoanalytic principles of inner conflict and repetition compulsion. Both Perel and Willi advocate the encounter between two different subjects. Willi approaches this through psychotherapeutic conflict analysis: he takes no sides but highlights stereotyped emotional and behavioural interactions. Perel's method is more pragmatic and provocative. Though inspired by psychoanalytic thought, her clinical focus lies primarily on mobilising desire, communication, and imagination. Whereas Willi shows why and where we become stuck, Perel shows how we might continue to desire even in or despite the familiar.

Jack the Lack

Perel's paradox ('Love enjoys knowing everything about you; desire needs mystery')[16] aligns with Jacques Lacan's fundamental insight that desire exists only through lack, distance, and the unknowability of the Other. Eroticism flourishes where there is room for projection, alterity, and not-knowing.[17] This resonates with Winnicott's concept of transitional space, where play, fantasy, and creativity can thrive.[18] Jessica Benjamin adds that vitality is possible only through recognising the other as an autonomous subject. Erotic desire is not fusion but a dialectic of proximity and difference.[19]

Willi analysed partner relationships as collusions: unconscious alliances in which partners take on complementary roles that echo unresolved childhood conflicts. Love is understood as the re-performance of the familiar, or the confirmation of what was already known within one's neurotic structure. The beloved is not the Other but a repetition of an internal drama. This analysis closely aligns with the Lacanian concept of *le partenaire symptôme*.[20] Here, the beloved partner is not simply an affective object but a symptomatic one; chosen because he or she uniquely activates and stabilises the subject's fantasy. Love is thus not merely 'falling for someone' but an unconscious choice: an investment in a partner who embodies the subject's internal conflict. The symptom in this context is not necessarily pathological but structural: a necessary construction that holds the subject together. The partner is not a symptom but, in Lacan's neologism, a *sinthome*: that which the subject requires to make its own dividedness bearable.[21] Love becomes a form of self-organisation through the other: fragile threads of a necessary attachment to one's own lack.

Perel and Willi both understand infidelity not merely as destructive but as expressive of underlying dynamics. For Perel, affairs are attempts to reconnect with a forgotten self; for Willi, they represent regressive escapes from stifling collusion. In Lacanian terms, infidelity often marks the moment when the existing symptom loses its stabilising power and a new partner-symptom imposes itself – another subject who activates a different fantasy.

Lacan's *le partenaire symptôme* adds that therapy entails confronting the impossibility of complete reciprocity. The partner is never a purely mirroring object but embodies something of one's own lack. Therapy, therefore, concerns less the resolution of conflict than the conscious bearing of the symptom embodied by the other. Perel, Willi, and Lacan together provide a rich, layered understanding of love as structure. Love is not the disappearance of boundaries but the endurance of difference. It is as much repetition as creation, as much symptom as desire. *Le partenaire symptôme* shows that we love where we are wounded, and that the other often becomes the bearer of what we lack. Erotic intelligence is thus the ability not to fill this lack but to live with it: playfully, imaginatively, and with desire.

Notes

1 Huxley, A. (1932/2007). *Brave new world*. New York: Vintage.
2 Freud, S. (1905/1953). *Three essays on the theory of sexuality* (J. Strachey, Trans.). In J. Strachey (Ed.), *The standard edition of the complete psychological works of Sigmund Freud* (Vol. 7, pp. 123–245). London: Hogarth Press.
3 Balint, M. (1965). *Primary love and psycho-analytic technique*. New York: Liveright.
4 Kernberg, O. F. (1995). *Love relations: Normality and pathology*. New Haven: Yale University Press.
5 Lacan, J. (1972–1973/1975). *Le Séminaire, Livre XX: Encore* (p. 13). Paris: Seuil.
6 Beckett, S. (1983). *Worstward ho* (p. 7). New York: Grove Press.
7 Lacan, J. (1964/1973). *Le Séminaire, Livre XI: Les quatre concepts fondamentaux de la psychanalyse* (p. 55). Paris: Seuil.
8 We were both born in Belgium in 1958, the year of the Brussels World Expo and the Atomium.
9 Perel, E. (2006). *Mating in captivity: Unlocking erotic intelligence*. New York: Harper Collins.
10 Winnicott, D. W. (1971). *Playing and reality*. London: Tavistock Publications.
11 Klein, M. (1946/1997). Notes on some schizoid mechanisms. In M. Klein, *Envy and gratitude and other works 1946–1963* (pp. 1–24). New York: Vintage.
12 Laplanche, J. (1999). *Essays on otherness*. London/New York: Routledge.
13 Perel, E. (2017). *The state of affairs: Rethinking infidelity*. New York: Harper Collins.
14 Lacan, J. (1958/2006). The direction of the treatment and the principles of its power. In *Écrits: The first complete edition in English* (B. Fink, Trans., pp. 489–542). New York: Norton.
15 Willi, J. (1975/1992). *Die Zweierbeziehung: Wirklichkeit und Illusion der Liebe* (10e druk). München: Piper.
16 Perel, E. (2006). *Mating in captivity: Unlocking erotic intelligence* (p. 37). New York, NY: HarperCollins.
17 Lacan, J. (1958/2006). The direction of the treatment and the principles of its power. In *Écrits: The first complete edition in English* (B. Fink, Trans., pp. 489–542). New York: Norton.

18 Winnicott, D. W. (1971). *Playing and reality*. London: Tavistock Publications.
19 Benjamin, J. (1988). *The bonds of love: Psychoanalysis, feminism, and the problem of domination*. New York: Pantheon.
20 Miller, J.-A. (2015). *Le partenaire-symptôme: L'orientation lacanienne (1997–1998)*. Paris: La Martinière/Le Champ freudien.
21 Lacan, J. (1975/2023). *Le Séminaire, livre XXIII: Le sinthome*. Paris: Seuil. For Lacan, the *sinthome* is the unique, personal way in which a subject secures structural support for its existence. It is a particular mode of knotting that holds together the three registers (the Real, the Symbolic, and the Imaginary) when the symbolic order falters. In that sense, it is not a symptom to be dissolved but an idiosyncratic solution: a stabilising fourth knot that prevents the subject from coming undone. With this shift, Lacan moves from the symptom as something to be interpreted to the *sinthome* as something one learns to live with. See Kinet, M. (2015). Het sinthoom als kunstgreep. *Tijdschrift voor Psychoanalyse*, *1*, 70–72.

20

Love Generations

Learning

Every generation must learn how to love again. What changes is not only the vocabulary of desire, but the very texture of intimacy: what bodies mean, how they touch, what they dare to want. My first erotic stimuli were very discreet: a squaw from a cowboy film emerging from a river wearing a wet chamois leather skirt, models in lingerie in my mother's *Trois Suisses* catalogue, my first glimpse of bare breasts on television, a pack of playing cards with topless pin-ups in my father's bedside table, pornographic magazines hidden under towels in the cupboard. It all built up very gradually, allowing my libido to grow slowly, which was also the pace of my actual practices in these matters. I sometimes wonder what would have happened if we had grown up under constant sexual bombardment.

From the baby boomers' post-war liberation to Generation Z's digital hesitancy, sexuality has been the mirror in which Western culture recognises its shifting anxieties and aspirations. Love is always historical, but its history is written in the language of the unconscious: that theatre where, as Freud said, there is no negation and no time.[1]

As a generational prototype, I myself was born into a world eager to forget. After the devastations of war, a new morality promised prosperity, family stability, and consumer fulfilment. Yet, beneath the clean surfaces of the 1950s lay a longing to break free from repression. Freud's discovery of the drives had long since unsettled bourgeois respectability, but it was only in the 1960s that sexuality became a political language. The pill, legalised abortion, and feminist consciousness did not simply liberate sex from reproduction; they transformed it into a declaration of autonomy. But the slogan *Make Love* was never purely erotic. It carried a utopian charge: the belief that freeing desire would free society itself. Foucault would later argue that sexuality became the privileged site of modern power: by speaking about sex, we imagined ourselves liberated, even as we remained caught in its discourse.[2] Still, we baby boomers experienced our awakening as an emancipation of the body from guilt and hierarchy. The naked body became a manifesto; nudity, a politics. Yet the psychoanalytic eye discerns ambivalence. Liberation remained haunted by the very repression it sought to

DOI: 10.4324/9781003728764-22

overcome. The Freudian 'return of the repressed' took the form of new compulsions (performance, seduction, authenticity) that bound subjects to a new invisible superego of pleasure. Love, once bound to duty, was now bound to freedom itself.

Those born between 1965 and 1980 (Generation X) inherited the promises of the sixties but grew up in their shadow. The sexual revolution had institutionalised itself: desire was no longer forbidden but required. Then came the AIDS crisis, transforming pleasure into risk. What had been utopian now demanded prophylaxis. The hippie's erotic optimism gave way to the nightclub's cynicism. Generation X developed an ironic relationship with intimacy. Influenced by postmodernism, they distrusted grand narratives, including that of romantic love. The condom replaced the ring as the symbol of responsibility. Pleasure was still sought, but always with a trace of anxiety. Lacan might have said that the *objet petit a* had migrated from the body to the screen: pornography became a mirror of alienation, a spectacle of desire detached from reciprocity.[3] In psychoanalytic terms, one might say this was a shift from *Eros* to *Thanatos*: from the creative union of drives to their self-destructive repetition. McDougall spoke of 'the theatre of the body': when language falters, the body acts.[4] In Generation X, the body oscillated between display and withdrawal, between MTV seduction and burnout. Love was still desired, but it was put in quotation marks.

Digits

Millennials, born between 1981 and 1996, came of age amidst digitalisation, globalisation, and the rhetoric of self-realisation. They were the first to live their erotic lives both online and offline. For them, sexuality became a form of identity work: a performative project of self-definition. The question was no longer simply whom one desired, but what that desire meant about oneself. The vocabulary of consent, diversity, and empowerment reshaped erotic discourse. The feminist and queer movements had made visible the structural asymmetries of desire; love was now negotiated through ethics. Yet the freedom to define oneself produced new anxieties. Illouz has shown how, under capitalism, emotional life becomes a marketplace of experiences: desire is managed, compared, and optimised. Tinder profiles and curated authenticity transformed the subject into both a lover and a brand.[5]

Psychoanalysis might read this as the triumph of the imaginary over the symbolic. The gaze (once the site of Lacan's *scopic drive*)[6] now returned as the selfie. Love was staged as self-representation. Behind this surface, many Millennials felt the erosion of depth, the fatigue of having to desire meaningfully. The command to 'be yourself' became another form of superegoic pressure: enjoy responsibly, desire correctly, love sustainably.

For Generation Z, born between 1997 and 2012, there is no distinction between the digital and the real. Their first erotic object was the screen; their first language of love, the emoji. They are both overexposed and under-touched. Pornography is ubiquitous yet unremarkable, its endless availability flattening difference and suspense. The Freudian fantasy, once a unique construction of the unconscious, is now algorithmically prefabricated.

This generation grew up amidst the #MeToo movement, climate anxiety, and the omnipresence of mental health discourse. Their sexuality is cautious, reflexive, and often virtual. 'Consent' has become not only a legal safeguard but also a moral ideal – a means of reclaiming control in a hyperconnected world. Yet, as Byung-Chul Han notes, the neoliberal subject of transparency tends to abolish mystery and, with it, desire itself.[7]

Love requires opacity, the not-knowing that invites projection, imagination, risk. In a culture of exposure, this opacity is vanishing. Generation Z experiences what might be called *jouissance fatigue*: overstimulated, yet under-moved. They seek authenticity through digital means that constantly betray it. Žižek would call this the 'interpassivity' of late capitalism: we outsource our enjoyment to the screen, letting devices desire for us.[8]

Psychoanalytically, the locus of desire has shifted again: from the interpersonal to the interfacial. The other no longer looks back; it scrolls. The mirror stage now unfolds within the algorithmic gaze. Love persists, but in the form of ghosting, lurking, and curated vulnerability.

The children of Millennials, born after 2013, are still forming their libidinal maps. Yet their environment already predicts a new topology of intimacy. They are raised amidst AI companions, virtual influencers, and parental surveillance. Their first attachments may not be to persons but to interfaces that simulate responsiveness without subjectivity.

If Freud's 'psychical apparatus' was once bounded by repression, the digital psyche of Generation Alpha is bounded by data. The algorithm anticipates their desires before they are conscious of them. What happens to sexuality when anticipation replaces fantasy? When the other's desire is already known, even manufactured, there is little room for the unconscious.

Still, psychoanalysis reminds us that desire cannot be programmed away. The unconscious will find its detours: in art, rebellion, withdrawal, or unexpected tenderness. Perhaps Generation Alpha will rediscover the erotic not as consumption but as encounter: the fragile, unpredictable space where love interrupts efficiency.

Yearning

Seen across these generations, Western sexuality and the arc of desire have moved from repression (Baby Boomers) to liberation (Boomers/X/X) to regulation (AIDS, consent) to identification (Millennials) to virtualisation (Gen Z/Z/Alpha). Each phase promises freedom but produces new constraints. The libido, like capital, reinvents its economies. Freud's dialectic of Eros and Thanatos remains applicable: the drive towards life continually risks self-exhaustion. Lacan reframed this as the endless circulation of desire around the void of lack. In every epoch, culture tries to fill that void -with pleasure, safety, identity, data- and in doing so, reproduces it. Love endures precisely because it fails.

The psychoanalytic question is therefore not 'how has sex changed?' but 'how does each generation defend itself against desire?' The Baby Boomers feared repression; Generation X feared contamination; Millennials feared insignificance; Generation Z fears exposure. In each case, the fantasy of control replaces the risk of encounter. Most poignant is the risk of no longer longing.

If contemporary subjects suffer less from repression than from exhaustion, as Han suggests, psychoanalysis must adapt its listening.[9] The modern symptom is not neurosis but depletion: a difficulty in sustaining desire when every object is instantly available. The task is no longer to liberate the libido but to protect its capacity for yearning. Love becomes a counter-cultural act. To love is to resist the algorithmic capture of desire; to reintroduce delay, ambiguity, and otherness. In the words of Jessica Benjamin, recognition is mutual only when we allow the other's difference to unsettle us.[10] Each generation must rediscover this art of being affected. The cultural history of sexuality thus reads like a psychoanalytic case: a patient oscillating between repression and compulsion, between fantasy and fatigue. The cure is not a return to innocence but a recovery of depth. Love remains the most subversive of forces because it reawakens the unconscious in an age that seems (or seeks) to abolish it.

Notes

1 Freud, S. (1915/1957). The unconscious (J. Strachey, Ed. & Trans.). In *The standard edition of the complete psychological works of Sigmund Freud* (Vol. 14, pp. 159–215). London: Hogarth Press.
2 Foucault, M. (1978). *The history of sexuality, Volume I: An introduction.* New York: Pantheon Books.
3 Miller, J.-A. (1997). *Lacan et la pornographie. La Cause freudienne, 36,* 7–18.
4 McDougall, J. (1989). *Théâtres du corps: Le psychosoma en psychanalyse.* Paris: Gallimard.
5 Illouz, E. (2007). *Cold intimacies: The making of emotional capitalism.* Cambridge: Polity Press.
6 Lacan, J. (1963/1973). *Le Séminaire, Livre XI : Les quatre concepts fondamentaux de la psychanalyse* (J.-A. Miller, Éd.). Paris: Seuil.
7 Han, B.-C. (2010/2015). *The burnout society* (E. Butler, Trans.). Stanford: Stanford University Press.
8 Žižek, S. (1999). *The ticklish subject: The absent centre of political ontology.* London/New York: Verso.
9 Han, B.-C. (2010/2015). *The burnout society* (E. Butler, Trans.). Stanford: Stanford University Press.
10 Benjamin, J. (1988). *The bonds of love: Psychoanalysis, feminism, and the problem of domination.* New York: Pantheon Books.

21

The Shadows of Love

Sacred Love?

Love is far from sacred. Like all things under the sun, its graceful appearance conceals many shadows. Upon closer inspection, it is invariably based, at least in part, on illusion and deceit. Beneath the cloak of love, more negative elements are consistently concealed. Oblative, selfless love is a chimaera, a fantasy held by some devout souls. More often, instinct and the pursuit of pleasure serve noble parts rather than noble purposes. Maturity, therefore, demands a measure of disillusionment about love. And yet, love and travel remain the most popular means of turning a dream into reality.

Love is not a given; it is the result of a developmental process, a struggle *to* love. It is a value to be attained, and it remains perpetually at risk. Platonists and Christians believe that love can deepen and grow throughout life, even as desire is expected to ebb more than flow. For them, love certainly includes pleasure, but it also endures pain. Care and concern for others are essential components. As we all know, not all love is equally pleasurable. Dependency and neediness, then, are at most forerunners of love, lacking true concern for the other. In such cases, declarations of love are transparently disguised *needs* for love. When the love object is expected to meet a more or less vital need, love becomes somewhat monstrous. It may stifle or even destroy the other. It is a kind of love experienced as a pursuit rather than support. It borders on hate, for it obstructs the path to autonomy and identity. Likewise, infantile drives are only precursors to love. The desires to suck or be suckled, to see or be seen, to lead or be led (while foundational elements) do not in themselves constitute love worthy of the name.

Those in love with themselves enjoy the benefit of few rivals. Related to this is the idea that it is not love that is blind, but self-love. The first passionate and captivating Gestalt that captures the child is its own mirror image. Its first two love objects are not only the mother but also the self. A mother's eyes are both the child's first mirror and (through their 'Reflections in a Golden Eye') the origin of a 'Golden I.'[1]

DOI: 10.4324/9781003728764-23

Actual Love

Thereafter, humans choose two types of love objects. The first involves figures who literally or figuratively offer nourishment, care, and protection: the so-called anaclitic object-choice. Many seeking marriage long for a nurturing mother figure. These partners can also be seen as accomplices in a joint escape from loneliness. The second possibility concerns figures chosen in the image of the self or of one's ideal: the narcissistic object choice. Freud's example is Leonardo da Vinci, who sought to love boys as he himself had been loved by his mother. Homophilia can also be regarded as a form of egophilia. In more modern terms, it concerns the twin, the soulmate, or the other-equal who confronts us as little as possible with (sexual) difference.

In practice, every actual love object is typically an alloy of these two poles. What emerges from this genealogy is that there is no absolute opposition between love of the other and love of the self. Inverting Rimbaud's famous phrase '*Je est un autre,*' we might say: '*L'autre est un je.*'[2]

According to a perhaps equally well-known phrase of Freud, the shadow of the object falls upon the ego. He inferred this from the observation that most lovers begin to resemble one another. Identifications with the lost beloved, as seen in mourning, can also be understood in this way. But we may also invert this formulation: the shadow of the ego falls upon the object. In love, there is always a relationship with the other, both as other and as self. This reciprocity, with its subtle dialectic of sameness and difference, is a defining trait of any loving relationship. The beloved is at once an incestuous object and an Ego-Ideal; the so-called incestuous desire expresses a longing to return to a shared, quasi-divine ideal state.[3]

Hateful Love

In *Drives and Their Vicissitudes*, Freud asserts that hate precedes love.[4] Hate is older than love, and the parent of love. When frustration makes a child aware of its dependency, hate and anger arise and henceforth accompany any revival of original narcissistic injuries. These feelings are integral to love. Only such negative emotions make separation and detachment possible. The tongue and lips may suffice for suckling, but teeth are needed for distance, for biting away the Other. Hate also contributes to recognising the other as other.

According to post-Freudian Donald Winnicott, our first experience of love is primitive. He calls it 'mouthlove'[5] – a ruthless love in which the other is drained and discarded. Tenderness only emerges from a developing capacity for concern. If all goes well, both love and the love object survive our early assaults. Gradually, the child becomes aware of the love object's alterity and subjectivity.

It was once thought that time would simplify love. It does not. It only reveals more clearly what in love cannot be repaired, and what, strangely, does not need to be.

From the perspective of Melanie Klein, many acts of love are reparative reaction-formations against aggressive or sadistic feelings and fantasies.[6] For her, love is primarily the result of guilt and the wish to make amends. In our earliest phase of life, 'evil' was situated outside of us. All inner tensions were attributed to a threatening external world. Only later do we arrive at what Klein calls the 'depressive position': an awareness that evil resides within rather than outside of us. This marks a kind of Cape of Good Hope, allowing us to take our fate into our own hands and to begin a lifelong task of repair.

The triumph of love over hate becomes the goal of a relentless inner struggle. Destructive drives are redirected towards nobler aims. Guilt feelings, remnants of a kind of original sin from our personal prehistory, foster a relational ethic of care. This leads to altruistic and friendly forms of love, where care for the object takes precedence. These types of love overcome sadistic impulses and primitive, devouring forms of attachment. Only then do we truly find fulfilment in our connections. In addition to the depressive position, the Oedipus complex plays a key role in civilisation. Its taboos – against incest and parricide – give rise to *philia*, the deep parental love that forges familial bonds. This love transcends its bodily roots and, as a sublimation of *eros*, relinquishes its sexual aim.

Maniac

Not every love brings solace. In the Greek concept of *mania*, love retains a mad, jealous, and malicious aspect. The lover desperately tries to preserve a sense of self-worth that only the partner can provide. Toxic behaviours such as stalking, dependency, and paranoid jealousy may result in violent attempts to possess the beloved exclusively. Stalking has been called an old behaviour but a new crime. It is the behaviour of the rejected 'lover' who pursues the beloved against their will. The lover bombards the beloved with flowers, floods them with...into ther private space...their most intimate feelings or parts. By meddling in every detail of her life, he enacts a fantasy of omnipotent control. Research shows that such stalkers are often men who suffered early disruptions in attachment. Rejection and loss may trigger this behaviour. Narcissistic and fusion fantasies that are frustrated or dismissed evoke shame and humiliation. These ignite a whirlwind of rage that both propels and explodes their 'love offensive.'

This is the macro-visible, adult variation on an infantile theme, where primitive and monstrous forms of 'love' reach their peak. It is a revival of sadistic and cannibalistic assaults on the (m)other. Rage and hatred are then the fallout of a once enchanting, but ultimately fragile bubble: gold-leaf-thin.

Notes

1 Kinet, M. (2005). Reflections in a golden I. In M. Kinet & L. Moyson (Red.), *Grootse patiënten, kleine therapeuten. Over psychotherapie en narcisme* (pp. 7–19). Antwerpen/Apeldoorn: Garant.
2 Rimbaud, A. (1871/1958). Lettre à Georges Izambard, 13/05/1871. In: *Œuvres*. Paris: Mercure.

3 Chasseguet-Smirgel, J. (1975). *L'idéal du moi* (pp. 305–306). Paris: Tchou.
4 Freud, S. (1915). Driften en hun lotgevallen. P.T.**2.** *Sigmund Freud Nederlandse Editie* (pp. 31–65). Amsterdam/Meppel: Boom.
5 Winnicott, D. W. (1963/1990). The development of the capacity for concern. In *The maturational process and the facilitating environment*. London: Karnac.
6 Klein, M. (1959/1975). Our adult world and its roots in infancy. In *The writings of Melanie Klein* (Vol. IV). London: Hogarth.

Unnatural Love

An Unusable Concept

Before Freud, and even today in common parlance, perversity is understood as a deviation from instinct. This instinct is conceived as a predetermined behaviour, innate to a particular species, and relatively unchangeable in its direction and object.[1] From this point of view, perversion is deemed unnatural. Whatever dictionary one consults, the term 'perversion' always carries the sense of turning upside down or inside out (Latin: *pervertere*), but typically in the direction of evil or wrong. It thus has a pejorative tone, evoking moral disapproval, disgust, or fear. When someone's behaviour is described as perverse, we usually intuit that it involves an 'improper' use of something otherwise legitimate. One shudders before the enjoyment presumed to fuel it.[2] That's why perversion is today a largely abandoned term. Psychiatry replaced it with *paraphilia*, cultural discourse prefers the more playful register of *kink*, and clinical practice increasingly avoids its moral weight. But the experience it names has not vanished. Beneath the glamour of contemporary erotic culture, beneath the choreography of consent and the commodity-aesthetic of desire, an older drama persists: the struggle between longing and law, fantasy and recognition, the body and its ghosts.

Nowadays, psychoanalysis no longer treats perversion as mere sexual deviance. It views it instead as a privileged lens through which to read fantasy and the subject's relation to the Other. What counts as 'perverse' shifts historically, but the psychic mechanisms Freud and colleagues described remain remarkably stable.[3] In an early (but meanwhile surpassed) view, the pervert simply enacts what the neurotic merely fantasises: no repression, only unbridled acting out. Already in a letter to Fliess, Freud hypothesised that perversion might be the negative of neurosis.[4] The pervert acts out what the neurotic represses. Neurotic shyness, stammering, and blushing are the negative images of perverse exhibitionism. In his classic psychoanalytic terminology, the notion of perversion is narrowed to the domain of sexuality.[5] It refers to a deviation from the standard sexual act, i.e. coitus culminating in orgasm through genital penetration between individuals of different sexes. One speaks of (implicitly sexual) perversion when orgasm only occurs through another sexual object, other bodily zones, or becomes compulsively dependent on

DOI: 10.4324/9781003728764-24

specific external conditions. In a brief and laconic formula, the pervert is someone who does not make love like most others.

Law

If neurosis is the primary field of psychoanalysis, and psychosis that of classical psychiatry, then perversity lies more broadly within the domain of the social, and at times even the legal norm. This norm, of course, varies across historical and/or cultural contexts. For example, homosexuality (‘*paederastia*’) was the highest form of love in ancient Greece, a mortal sin in Christianity, a degenerative condition in nineteenth-century psychiatry, and, since the 1970s, has been considered one form of sexuality among others.[6]

In psychiatry, under the influence of changing cultural climates, the term ‘perversion’ was replaced in the 1980s by ‘paraphilia.’ This term limits the field of sexual anomalies to practices involving coercion, based on the absence of a freely consenting partner, or having a fetishistic character. Psychoanalysis, too, evolves with its time. Some authors in a 1986 special issue of *The International Journal of Psycho-Analysis* argue that perversion applies only when the subject, by placing something between themselves and the other, fails to recognise the other as both person and Other, keeping them at a distance and using them purely as an object of drive satisfaction.[7] Sexual contact in situations of unfreedom and unequal dependence, such as child sexual abuse, then becomes a prototypical case of perversion.[8] Conversely, a relationship marked by intimacy and reciprocity shouldn’t be called perverse.

Psychoanalysis now considers perversion not as an exotic pathology but as a specific solution to psychic conflict. The psychodynamic is the only theoretical model to grasp its ‘reason’. Freud’s foundational insights were thereby transformed by Melanie Klein, Jacques Lacan, Robert Stoller, Joyce McDougall, Otto Kernberg, and Sergio Benvenuto. Although each approaches perversity from a different angle (developmental, structural, relational, ethical), together they reveal a complex psychic organisation in which sexuality, aggression, disavowal, trauma, and symbolic law are tightly interwoven. The contemporary preference for *kinky sex* may obscure its ‘gravity’, but the psychic economies that animate it are ancient, and its dynamics remain unmistakably psychoanalytic.

Infantile Sexuality

Freud approached so-called normal human sexuality through a study of perversions and infantile psychosexual development. In his analysis of various manifestations of perversion, he found reasons to challenge traditional views.[9] Before him, childhood was the last refuge of imagined innocence. It was assumed that children possessed no sexual drive and that sexuality would only emerge in puberty, triggered by bodily maturation. It was believed to manifest as an irresistible attraction between the sexes, culminating in intercourse or related acts. But Freud saw in children a vast experimental field: their play, curiosity, impulses, and confusions revealed that sexuality is not instinctual but creative, polymorphous, and fundamentally errant. It obeys no natural teleology. Genital sexuality, far from being the norm, is a cultural achievement that depends on repression, sublimation, and the acceptance of loss.

Freud, therefore, reconceptualised human sexuality not as instinctual but as unnatural or 'cultural.'[10] The frequency of perverse behaviour, as well as the persistence of perverse tendencies underlying neurotic symptoms or integrated into sexual activity, led Freud to conclude that the disposition to perversity is not rare, but part of the normal constitution: the child's polymorphously perverse disposition. Freud emphasised the wild, barbaric nature of this sexuality: a raw, infantile sexuality that draws upon all imaginable objects and aims for its satisfaction, underpinned by the infantile sexual theories he would describe elsewhere.[11] The child's drive does not know what is normal or natural; it seeks satisfaction wherever the body opens a path. After all, infantile sexuality still lacks the prohibition against incest and the possibilities of repression and sublimation.

Adult genital sexuality, on the other hand, is a fragile cultural achievement, not the biological norm. It can readily change shape in response to context and circumstances. Therefore, he re-imagined sexuality as a field of fluid impulses rather than a fixed biological function. Desire, he argued, is never purely reproductive but profoundly imaginative, driven by fantasy and its transformations. The 'perversions' he catalogued (e.g., voyeurism, fetishism, sadism, masochism) were less pathologies than mirrors of the creative distortions that make erotic life possible. In every lover's attachment, a trace of these archaic formations persists; the pervert merely renders them (more) visible.

Love, in its purest intensity, often reveals itself where the natural order falters. The so-called 'unnatural' forms of love (perverse, deviant, transgressive) are not foreign to the human condition but its encrypted truth. Freud saw perversion not as a moral deviation but as a structural possibility inherent in all desire: the child's polymorphous perversity never entirely disappears; it merely retreats beneath the veneer of civilisation. To love, then, is always to flirt with the forbidden, to touch that point where the drive resists domestication. Freud thus rejected the classical psychiatric view of perversion as degenerative or bestial. He instead saw it as a fixation. Against the social convention's normative standards, Freud set a different (amoral) norm: that of developmental organisation. Genital organisation establishes normality by subordinating partial and polymorphous sexuality to genital coitus. In a paradoxical sense, this norm is more absolute than the preceding moral standards, as genital organisation is supposed to transcend historical and cultural variation.

Castration

In the aforementioned letter to Fliess, Freud had already proposed a tripartite structure of hysteria, paranoia, and perversion.[12] In later writings, he gradually developed this more structural interpretation of perversion, characterised (not by repression or foreclosure but) by disavowal (of castration). This disavowal, or *Verleugnung*, denotes the simultaneous knowing and not-knowing of sexual difference. Through a study of fetishism,[13] in which castration anxiety results in this simultaneous recognition and denial Freud arrived at his final text on the matter: *The Splitting of the Ego in the Process of Defence*[14] Beyond the manifest and outward phenomena, the Freudian view became that perversion is an attempt to short-circuit the multiple effects of castration and, in a concealed manner, to restore the bond with the infantile incestuous objects within the perverse scenario. Perversion serves a defensive function, marked by a distinct intrapsychic organisation and psychodynamic mechanisms. It yields sexual satisfaction while simultaneously providing a feeling of safety by denying castration anxiety. This lends the perverse act its ritualistic and compulsive character.

All this is nowhere clearer than in fetishism, where the fetish becomes a substitute for the missing maternal phallus. Thanks to disavowal, the fetishist both acknowledges and denies castration: a double bookkeeping that becomes the hallmark of perversity. The child denies the absence of a penis in the girl[15] and instead believes in the phallic mother (or, in later Lacanian terms, the (M) Other without lack). This belief is present in all neurotics, but in the pervert it is simultaneously preserved and renounced. These two opposing positions can coexist thanks to a defensive 'splitting of the ego' (*Ich-Spaltung*). In this view, perversion is not only the result of fixation but of a specific position taken towards sexual difference or castration. Also, perversion is no longer simply exotic sexual behaviour. It is a fixation on infantile modes of satisfaction. It is a defence against castration anxiety. It creates a scenario that restores the illusion of omnipotence. It implies a denial of the Law rather than its absence. The perverse subject pays dearly for his little enjoyment, because they obey a rigid, compulsive scenario in which the partner becomes a function rather than a subject, while the pervert themself is driven by fear as much as by pleasure. That is why Freud called perverts pitiful souls who pay a heavy price for limited satisfaction.[16]

The Death Drive

It is well known that Freud's theory revolves primarily around the paternal figure. The primordial mother or the mother-environment is largely neglected in classical Freudian theory. Freud idealises the mother–child dyad, using it as the basis for myths of heaven and paradise.[17] Furthermore, there is no room in his thinking for a mother who is *not* good-enough. And yet, if fantasies of paradise stem from a nostalgia for the maternal breast, then representations of hell must likewise derive from this archaic developmental stage. One is reminded of Hieronymus Bosch's universe, with the God/Devil Baby as encountered in Melanie Klein's child analyses.[18]

Whereas Freud placed the drama of sexuality within the Oedipal triangle, Melanie Klein turned towards an earlier, even more turbulent landscape: the infant's relation to the first (part-) objects. For her, the seeds of later perversion lie not primarily in paternal prohibition but in the earliest anxieties of fragmentation, envy, annihilation, and dependence. The infant, caught between gratitude and aggression, forms internal objects that can live on as persecutors, saviours, or tyrants. Klein's view lends perversion a darker register. The perverse act becomes not simply a deviation of desire but an enactment of omnipotent control, a warding-off of dependency, a defensive triumph over internal terrors. Sexuality here is tinged with the death drive: aggression intrudes into erotic life, turning excitement into a weapon against the dreaded collapse of the self. Kleinian thought takes Freud's warring eros and thanatos with utmost seriousness. In the schizoid-paranoid position, aggression is projected outward, producing persecutory objects; in the depressive position, guilt and reparation become possible. The more severe perversions crystallise around distortions in the mother-child relationship during these early developmental stages.[19] They argue that perversions arise when mothers are not good-enough, speak of a premature emergence of genital feelings as a defence against the terror of pregenital impulses, or interpret the fetish as a failed transitional object.[20] For them, the perverse act does not primarily serve sexual gratification. It expresses attacks on the maternal object, a denial of dependency, omnipotent control over internal persecutors, and a corruption of sexuality by the death drive. Where Freud centres castration, Klein emphasises primitive anxieties of annihilation. From this perspective, perversion is not so much a sexual aberration as a brutal manifestation of thanatos, which in the therapeutic setting may lead to a negative therapeutic reaction or even the perversion of the transference itself. In the consulting room, the patient attempts to control, punish, or seduce the analyst to ward off psychic collapse.[21]

Benign vs Malign

Inspired by Ego Psychology and Kleinian thought, Otto Kernberg approaches perversion through his model of personality organisations.[22] Although he continues to regard the disavowal of castration as the foundational principle of perversions, for him, severe sexual perversions are typically embedded in borderline or pathological narcissistic structures. Their chaotic and multiple (i.e. in his classification: non-rigid!) perverse fantasies and acts involve unstable and promiscuous heterosexual and homosexual object relations wherein sadomasochistic tendencies predominate. His framework proves particularly relevant in forensic psychiatry, where certain perverse structures border on psychopathy. He distinguishes sharply between what he considers sexual variations or *benign kink* (such as consensual SM) and pathological perversion that is rooted in entitlement and lack of empathy. What distinguishes them is not the act but the *personality* behind it: the absence of empathy, the flattening of the other into a part-object, the ritualised repetition of cruelty. Where Klein highlights primitive anxieties, Kernberg reveals the characterological scaffolding that allows certain perverse patterns to become a fixed mode of relating.[23]

Structural Perversion

As is well known, Jacques Lacan claimed a direct lineage from Freud.[24] He reframes the entire field by completely removing perversion from the realm of behaviour. Its core mechanism is the *disavowal of castration*: 'I know very well, but all the same…' The core of the perverse question is complex, so I will circle around it several times in order to grasp it from every possible angle.

Perversion, for Lacan, is one of three linguistic or subjective positions (alongside neurosis and psychosis) in relation to the big Other and its lack.[25] What typifies perversion is the simultaneity and reversibility of yes and no, recognition and denial of castration. He elevates perversion to one of the essential modalities of psychic functioning: a kind of provocation of the Law, which is thereby disavowed. In Lacan's view, perversion is defined neither by acts nor preferences but by a position vis-à-vis the big Other. The neurotic wonders: *Che Vuoi?*[26] What does the Other want of me? The psychotic forecloses the Other entirely. The pervert takes it upon himself to *stage* what the Other is presumed to want.[27] In Lacan's view, the pervert recognises the law but subverts it. He transgresses the Law within the parameters of a self-fashioned morality. He imposes his own stance on pleasure and enjoyment upon the other. The relationship between partners in the perverse scenario is not mediated by the Law but is short-circuited by a *contract*.

In his famous 1963 essay *Kant avec Sade*, he continues his reasoning. There, Lacan equates Evil (in Sade's sense) with Good (in Kant's).[28] He argues that perverse structure is characterised by the subject's desire to become an object of enjoyment for the Other. The Law is meanwhile ridiculed, and what fuels the subject is an unconscious wish to dissolve into absolute evil and self-annihilation. In Lacanian terms, the perverse subject, through his act, stages the completeness of the big Other, identifying with the imaginary object of the mother's desire. He *plays* the missing piece of the Other. The pervert feels no guilt because he assumes the role of pure *instrument* for the whim of the big Other. He is not responsible for what he does; he merely carries out the will of a higher necessity. He even obeys the Law to the point of obscenity, revealing its underside. In this structure, guilt evaporates because the perverse subject believes he merely serves a higher mandate. The partner becomes a function, a cypher within the subject's script; reciprocity collapses; enjoyment is pushed past pleasure, towards the realm of excess that Lacan calls *jouissance*. This is the scandal of perversion: not its acts but its ethics: a dedication to sustaining the Other's enjoyment as if it were a sacred duty! The encounter with the perverse act confronts the neurotic, on the other hand, with his own inner dividedness, generating both horror and fascination. Recall the earlier point: the presumed surplus enjoyment attributed to the pervert by the non-pervert.

The neurotic *imagines* absolute enjoyment: in death, madness, or supreme bliss. The pervert does not imagine; he *seeks* it. He aims to capture absolute enjoyment. According to Juan-David Nasio, he may come closest to this enjoyment, but in a false manner: he *imitates* its gesture.[29] The perverse act is not transgression but service: the pervert sacrifices himself. Perversion is not the absence of morality but its inverted form: a form of devotion to the Law that both obeys and transgresses it. The pervert knows the Law exists, yet acts 'as if' it does not. This creates a space in which enjoyment and prohibition intertwine. The pleasure of the fetishist, for instance, depends on maintaining the illusion that the maternal lack can be denied, that the phallus is still present, displaced onto a substitute object.[2] What appears as pathology thus defends the subject against the unbearable anxiety of castration. The partner is not a person but a function, instrumentalised as a puppet in the scenario; enjoyment (*jouissance*) overrides pleasure, leading towards an ecstatic limit. The perverse scenario severs sexuality from reciprocity and places it in a circuit of mastery, submission, or fetishistic substitution whose aim is to sustain the illusion of an uncastrated (M)Other.

An Erotic Form of Hatred

In contrast to this (possibly rather abstract) aetiology, Robert Stoller returns to biography and unveils another truth: perversion is often a triumph over trauma. Many perverse scenarios, he argues, originate in childhood experiences of humiliation, intrusion, or emotional violation. The perverse script becomes a symbolic reversal of this early injury: the subject eroticises what once wounded him, transforming passive helplessness into active mastery. Hence, his famous formula: perversion is the erotic form of hatred.[30]

According to Stoller, perversion is not just a variant of sexual preference, but functions as a *ritual* in which the subject (in fantasy or deed) takes revenge on the person who once hurt him or her. The erotic component masks and camouflages the underlying hatred and resentment. Sexual arousal serves to conceal hatred and to express it, meaning that in the perversion one seeks not only sexual excitement but also revenge and mastery, all in a disguised form.[31] Another crucial element is scene construction: perverse acts are usually performed within rigid, carefully staged scenarios. This gives the subject maximum control over the situation, which is the opposite of the early traumatic experience in which the victim found themselves. Control is the *sine qua non* of perverse acts.[32] The pleasure is intense because it is soaked with victory. Hatred is disguised as arousal; humiliation becomes an instrument rather than a threat. Even masochism, in Stoller's reading, contains a paradoxical control: by choosing the conditions of one's own degradation, one avoids the chaos of unchosen pain. Stoller thus exposes the revenge woven into many perverse fantasies: the other is not sought for intimacy but used as a screen upon which an old wound is replayed and re-fashioned.

Stoller closely examines how perversion is staged through rigid scenarios. These can take various forms and are distinguished into sadomasochistic scripts, voyeuristic and exhibitionistic scripts, and fetishistic scripts.[33] For example, a person who was repeatedly humiliated as a child by a controlling mother will develop a sadomasochistic scenario in which sexual arousal depends on humiliating oneself or being humiliated. In the sadistic position, he can control and humiliate the other person in order to gain mastery over his former helplessness. In the masochistic position, he wants to humiliate himself in order to have control over the moment and form of the humiliation (paradoxical control).

Someone who was emotionally neglected by important others as a child may develop a perverse tendency towards exhibitionism: by shamelessly exposing themselves, the lack of *being seen* is finally compensated for in fantasy, and feelings of revenge are activated (others are embarrassed). A similar mechanism applies to voyeurism: by secretly observing, one seeks revenge for early experiences of exclusion, with a sense of superior control.

In fetishism (in which, e.g., shoes, leather, or latex play an important role), a fear of sexual and emotional intimacy is often replaced by a fetish object that isolates the affect. Stoller points out, for example that in some cases the choice of fetish object can be traced back to a scene of trauma or sexual confusion in childhood: e.g. a child who became fascinated by the aggressor's shoes during a traumatic event.

The resulting sexual scenario is a meticulously controlled reconstruction of that trauma, transformed (like children's play) from passive to active helplessness into mastery. Central to perversion is stereotypy of the script; perverse acts are rigid, theatrical, ritualistic. The perverse subject is 'in control': they determine every detail to prevent re-traumatisation. Pleasure is generated by triumph over the original injury, and sexual arousal is a camouflage, disguising hostility. Even from oneself. Examples include sadistic domination as a reversal of childhood powerlessness, masochistic self-abandonment as paradoxical control, or fetishistic enactments tied unconsciously to early scenes of confusion or shame.

Before concluding, I will offer some reflections inspired by Joyce McDougall and Sergio Benvenuto, whose views each provide a valuable supplement.

Neosexuality

In her *Plea for a Measure of Abnormality*, McDougall argues that the structural trinity of neurosis, psychosis, perversion (that was already proposed by Freud and further elaborated by Lacan) is too rigid to account for sexual deviations linked to various narcissistic disorders.[34] Drawing on both classical theory and her rich clinical sensibility, she proposed that many contemporary sexual deviations are neither structural perversions nor pathologies of hatred, but 'neosexualities' and sexual addictions: total psychic organisations that defend against fragmentation.[35] For her, perversion is a drama of the self. It may serve to maintain the fragile cohesion of the self and to defend against the collapse of psychic structure.[36] The perverse act is a play, a drama, a scenario through which unbearable affects are transformed into erotic intensity. Sexuality functions as an emotional analgesic or as an operator of cohesion. Many so-called perverts are dealing with narcissistic fragility rather than the disavowal of castration. She identifies three illusions served by perverse symptoms. First of all: castration doesn't exist. The law is empty, and sexual difference is denied. Second: sadism causes no harm because aggression is magically/sexually neutralised. Third: feelings of inner deadness are kept at bay by eroticism, warding off depression and emotional emptiness. In a way, McDougall thus softens

Stoller's emphasis on hatred and Kernberg's stress on primitive destructiveness. She sees perversion as a creative attempt to ensure psychic survival, not merely as pathology.

Like sexual fantasies, sexual deviations have for her an archaic underlying meaning, veiled in an eroticised scenario that integrates multiple themes and psychodynamic functions into a coherent whole. When one refrains from focusing solely on sexual behaviour and instead considers the personality as a whole, perverse sexuality appears as but one expression of a complex psychic state involving anxiety, inhibition, depression, and narcissistic disturbance. Perversion, or neosexuality, represents a total organisation that meets numerous intrapsychic needs, which renders the scenario stringent, compulsive, and rigid. The inventor of the neosexual script determines all the rules and assigns the role or function the partner must fulfil, including the idealised or despised elements they must embody, often revolving around a playful enactment of castration. Many perverts use sexuality as an opiate. The partner is denied as a separate individual and becomes a drug or a container for dangerous, split-off parts, which are managed at a distance through erotic control.

Caritas

Finally, Sergio Benvenuto, an Italian psychoanalyst and philosopher, offers a renewed and ethically attuned perspective on perversion. He reframes the conversation from behavioural definitions to the ethical dimension of sexual relations.[37] He argues that perversion arises when the subjectivity of the other is instrumentalised for one's own pleasure, without mutual recognition of the other as subject. Perversion, in this view, is not a moral failing but a strategy to transform suffering, such as exclusion or jealousy, into enjoyment by manipulating the other as a subject. A sexual act becomes perverse when the partner's interiority and subjectivity are completely disregarded, when suffering is reconverted into enjoyment, and there is no reciprocity whatsoever. Benvenuto calls this the *ethical failure* at the heart of perversion. It is the collapse of caritas, of mutual care, and of its substitution by unilateral mastery. His view echoes Stoller's emphasis on humiliation, yet emphasises the relational field rather than the trauma-derived scenario. Benvenuto's theory helps explain why consensual kink (even extreme forms) may not necessarily be perverse in the psychoanalytic sense. Reciprocity, negotiation, and recognition of the other's desire are intact.

To bring all the disparate elements that have been discussed together, here is a succinct clinical case description where there is *cuckolding* instead of holding.

Sammy

Sammy is a professional military man in his mid-forties who presents with anxiety and depression, but above all with sudden outbursts of rage in which his wife receives heavy blows. He states from the outset that he experienced no difficulties during the first 7 years of his life. He was raised primarily by his grandmother, with whom he felt safe and loved. By contrast, he has always felt unwanted by his parents. His mother had hoped for a daughter and was never able to accept him. When he was seven, a younger brother was born, whom he says was always her 'god.' He describes his mother as a selfish woman who exploited everything and everyone, and by whom he feels abandoned, betrayed, and robbed. His father was either absent or aggressive and violent. On several occasions, Sammy received punches to the face, losing multiple teeth as a result. Eventually, he pretended that none of it affected him. He links this to a later pattern in which he wages war against the entire world, like the Joker in the eponymous film.[38]

From a young age, he was frequently confronted with his father's pornographic videos. He was particularly fascinated and aroused by women with a penis. He became overstimulated and refers to himself as a 'hot bull,' while simultaneously doubting his gender identity: 'I feel as if I'm in the wrong body.' From adolescence onwards, he would put on women's clothes and masturbate in front of the mirror. In those moments, he felt both male and female. Although he did well in school, he was permitted to attend only until age fifteen. He was then forced into an apprenticeship, and all the money he earned thereafter had to be handed over to his parents. He joined the army and led a highly promiscuous and alcohol-fuelled life until he met his current wife. He moved in with her parents and found once again a measure of peace and stability. They have been together for more than 20 years and have three children, for whom he tries to care as best he can.

He soon persuaded his wife to accompany him to swinger clubs, and the couple rapidly moved towards what is known as 'cuckolding.' Sammy wanted his wife to have sex with other men in his presence, after which he himself would have intercourse with her. One of their children was, remarkably, conceived by one of these partners, who still visits several times a year on friendly terms. 'I want it that way too,' Sammy remarks. Over the course of therapy, it becomes clear that the perverse scenario revolves around motives such as jealousy, humiliation, and exclusion. In these situations, he is at once highly anxious and intensely aroused.

Even during the marriage, Sammy has frequently been unfaithful and adulterous. He claims to have been permanently in fight mode and only began to struggle severely after infidelity on the part of his wife. Since then, various triggers can provoke a 'primal rage' that suddenly takes hold. At times, 'everything goes black' before his eyes, and he completely loses control. He suffers from this himself and shows a genuine commitment to understanding this inner monster and thereby taming it. In an initial house drawing (made at the start of treatment), we observed a completely black, isolated house. Cracks run through it everywhere. A bolt of lightning splits the building in two. Beneath the house, there is a star-shaped crater, the result of an explosion. The roof appears to sit loose on the walls. Windows and doors are shuttered. From the first floor, bloody tears are flowing, and the jagged path leading to the door is also red with blood.

A Perverse Conclusion

Perversion is not the province of the monstrous few. It reveals something intimate about human love: our desire to master loss, deny separation, reverse pain, and serve an Other whose demands remain opaque. Whether understood through Klein's death-driven hatred, Lacan's structural disavowal, Stoller's traumatic revenge, McDougall's self-stabilising illusions, Kernberg's pathological aggression, or Benvenuto's ethical collapse, perversion ultimately exposes the fault-line where love and the drive intersect. Even in its modern, stylised form as 'kinky love,' it carries the same ancient tensions: tenderness interwoven with cruelty, dependence masked by dominance, vulnerability eroticised into control.

After all, the perverse act is not simply an expression of impulse but a form of communication, an attempt to tell the truth of one's desire when language fails. The 'unnatural' lover is thus not merely transgressive but profoundly relational, trapped in a choreography that both conceals and reveals his longing for reciprocity. When words fail, the body speaks. The script is rigid because it protects against psychic collapse. The roles are fixed because they originate in scenes too fragile to risk improvisation. Beneath apparent cruelty often lies a plea for recognition: see me where I could not be seen; hear me where I was silenced; hold me where I once shattered. Perversion dramatises the human effort to reconcile love and the drive. Where love seeks union, the drive insists on repetition and excess. Love addresses a subject, whereas the drive circles an object. Perversion, through its ritualised gestures, sustains this contradiction. It transforms the impossibility of fusion into a form of play, a space where the body speaks what the ego cannot articulate. In a culture obsessed with authenticity and consent, this ambivalence unsettles us, yet it also reminds us that love is never innocent. Even the most 'normal' forms of affection conceal a perverse kernel, a residue of childhood's unregulated desire.

To speak of unnatural love is not to condemn but to illuminate. It reminds us that desire is never purely natural, never free of its history. It reveals the fault line where tenderness meets aggression, where dependency becomes domination, and where fantasy unsettles reality. Every act of love may carry a shadow. Every gesture of care may have a trace of cruelty. Every desire risks a descent into the uncanny. That's why, referring to Paul Verhaeghe's award-winning *On Being Normal and Other Disorders*,[39] we arrive somewhat wryly on a perverse conclusion: to love 'naturally' may be the greatest perversion of all.

Notes

1 Tinbergen, N. (1951/1991). *The study of instinct: With a new preface*. Oxford: Oxford University Press.
2 Kinet, M. (2002). Onnatuurlijk. Verkennende gedachten over perversie. In M. Kinet & M. Thys (Eds.), *Liefdesverklaringen. Over perversie, liefde en passie* (pp. 25–32). Leuven/Leusden: Acco.
3 Kinet, M. (2006). *Freud & Co in de psychiatrie. Klinisch-psychotherapeutisch perspectief* (Psychoanalytisch Actueel, 3). Antwerpen/Apeldoorn: Garant.

4 Freud, S. (1896/1985). Letter to Wilhelm Fliess, 1 January 1896. In J. M. Masson (Ed. & Trans.), *The complete letters of Sigmund Freud to Wilhelm Fliess, 1887–1904* (p. 215). Cambridge: Harvard University Press.
5 Laplanche, J. en Pontalis, J.-B. (1967). *Vocabulaire de la psychanalyse*. Paris: PUF and Plon, M., & Roudinesco, E. (1997). *Dictionnaire de la Psychanalyse*. Paris: Fayard.
6 Boswell, J. (1980). *Christianity, social tolerance, and homosexuality*. Chicago: University of Chicago Press.
7 Glasser, M. (1986). Identification and its vicissitudes as observed in the perversions. *International Journal of Psycho-Analysis, 67*, 9–17.
8 McDougall, J. (1986). Identifications, neoneeds and neosexualities. *International Journal of Psycho-Analysis, 67*, 19–33.
9 Freud, S. (1905/1953 o.c.). Three essays on the theory of sexuality (J. Strachey, Ed. & Trans.). In J. Strachey (Ed.), *The standard edition of the complete psychological works of Sigmund Freud* (Vol. 7, pp. 125–243, p. 159). London: Hogarth Press.
10 Freud, S. (1915/2001). *Instincts and their vicissitudes*. In J. Strachey (Ed. & Trans.), *The standard edition of the complete psychological works of Sigmund Freud* (Vol. 14, pp. 111–140). London: Vintage.
11 In my last essay the similarity between infantile and bonobo sexuality will become obvious.
12 Freud, S. (1896/1985). Letter to Wilhelm Fliess, 1 January 1896. In J. M. Masson (Ed. & Trans.), *The complete letters of Sigmund Freud to Wilhelm Fliess, 1887–1904* (pp. 207–210). Cambridge, MA: Harvard University Press.
13 Freud, S. (1927/2001). *Fetishism*. In J. Strachey (Ed. & Trans.), *The standard edition of the complete psychological works of Sigmund Freud* (Vol. 21, pp. 149–157). London: Vintage.
14 Freud, S. (1938/1988). De splitsing van het Ik in het afweerproces. *Nederlandse Editie: Psychoanalytische Theorie 3* (pp. 249–254). Meppel/Amsterdam: Boom.
15 Freud, S. (1923/1988/1985). De genitale organisatie bij het kind. *Nederlandse Editie: Klinische Beschouwingen 3* (pp. 73–80). Meppel/Amsterdam: Boom.
16 Freud, S. (1919/1985). Een kind wordt geslagen. *Nederlandse Editie: Klinische Beschouwingen 3* (p. 23). Meppel/Amsterdam: Boom.
17 See Freud's emphasis on the paternal law in *Totem and Taboo* (1913/1955), his acknowledgment that the feminine and the maternal environment remained under-theorised in the *New Introductory Lectures* (1932/1964), and his discussion of religious paradise fantasies as regressions to the original mother–child unity in *The Future of an Illusion* (1927/1961) and *Civilization and its Discontents* (1930/1961).
18 Kinet, M. (1996). Weerzien met. Melanie Klein. *Tijdschrift voor Psychotherapie, 3*, 197–211.
19 Bach, S. (1994). *The language of perversion and the language of love*. New York: Jason Aronson. Khan, M. M. R. (1979). *Alienation in perversions*. London: The Hogarth Press.
20 Greenacre, Ph. (1969). The fetish and the transitional object. *The Psychoanalytic Study of the Child, 24*, 144–164.
21 Britton, R. (1998). *Belief and imagination*. London: Routledge.
22 Kernberg, O. F. (1975). Borderline states and pathological narcissism. New York: Jason Aronson; Kernberg, O. F. (1984). *Severe personality disorders: Psychotherapeutic strategies*. New Haven, CT: Yale University Press.
23 Kernberg, O. F. (1992/2004). *Aggression in personality disorders and perversions*. New Haven: Yale University Press.
24 Lacan, J. (1955). La chose freudienne ou sens du retour à Freud en psychanalyse. In *Ecrits* (pp. 401–436). Paris: Seuil.
25 Lacan, J. (1964/1973). *Le Séminaire, livre XI: Les quatre concepts fondamentaux de la psychanalyse (1964)* (J.-A. Miller, Éd.). Paris: Seuil.

26 Kinet, M. (2025). Che Vuoi? Epiloog in enkele contrapunten. In M. Hebbrecht & J. De Vleminck (Red.), *Verleiding en vertaling. Het enigma van de seksualiteit* (pp. 173–189). Antwerpen/'s Hertogenbosch: Gompel&Svacina.
27 Lacan, J. (1962–1963/2004). *Le Séminaire, livre X: L'angoisse (1962–1963)* (J.-A. Miller, Éd.). Paris: Seuil.
28 Lacan, J. (1963/1966). Kant avec Sade. In *Ecrits*. Paris: Seuil.
29 Nasio, J. -D. (1992). *Cinq leçons sur la théorie de Jacques Lacan*. Paris: Rivages.
30 Stoller, R. J. (1975). *Perversion: The erotic form of hatred*. New York: Pantheon Books.
31 Stoller, R. J. (1975). *Perversion: The erotic form of hatred* (p. xxii). New York: Pantheon Books.
32 Stoller, R. J. (1975). *Perversion: The erotic form of hatred* (pp. 155–156). New York: Pantheon Books.
33 Stoller, R. J. (1985). *Observing the erotic imagination*. New Haven: Yale University Press.
34 McDougall, J. (1978/1980). *Plea for a measure of abnormality*. New York: International Universities Press.
35 McDougall, J. (1986). Identifications, neoneeds and neosexualities. *International Journal of Psycho-Analysis*, *67*, 19–33.
36 McDougall, J. (1985). *The many faces of Eros: A psychoanalytic exploration of human sexuality* (p. 102). New York: Norton.
37 Benvenuto, S. (2018). *What are perversions?: Sexuality, ethics, psychoanalysis*. London/New York: Routledge.
38 Phillips, T. (Director). (2019). *Joker* [Film]. Warner Bros. Pictures.
39 Verhaeghe, P. (2008/2020). *On being normal and other disorders*. London/New York: Routledge.

23

Passion Victims

Vogue

Passion is in vogue. Passion for travel, for reading, for cinema. Passion for scouring antique markets, for Indian cuisine, for growing cherry tomatoes. When it comes to passion, there seems to be something for everyone – although not every passion is equally trendy. For instance, the passion for raising children enjoys far less appeal than that for steamy sex. Passion appears to be an option one can choose, and strangely, it is a vital accessory if one wishes to avoid being labelled a dreary bore or nerd.

If we abstract from such trivial forms, the hallmark of passion is its excessiveness. Ecstasy and excess appear to be the hard, impenetrable, and unfathomable grain around which the pearl of passion forms. In the realm of love, passion primarily refers to intensity and turbulence. As a noun, it can be considered an extreme form of infatuation in which one is seized not by the tangible, physical other, but by the elusive, the absolute. It is the magnification of a prolonged infatuation that cannot transform into any other form of loving and that leads to both physical and mental exhaustion. It is a searing, consuming fire, in which one wishes to die of not being able to die from love: *mourir de ne pas mourir*, as the mystics once put it.[1]

The impassioned subject becomes fascinated by a love object that overturns their entire lifeworld, to which they are bound with a dependency bordering on addiction. We are reminded of Jean-Paul Sartre's words: '*Dans la fascination il n'y a qu'un objet géant dans un monde désert*.'[2] For the fascinated lover, there exists only a colossal object in a desolate world. What is most striking in passion is that the lover does not truly seem to find joy in the presence of the beloved. Yet according to Spinoza, what characterises love is precisely the joy that something simply is as it is[3] – for instance, the warmth that overtakes us at the sight of our beloved asleep.

Love is always somewhat mingled with desire – the desire to caress, to cherish, to draw the other close. But love transcends this desire. In passion, by contrast, desire proves stronger than love. More specifically, it is the love for the desire of the love-object that outweighs the love for the object itself. In passion, love contracts into mere desire. Difference and lack are not only tolerated but sought out, cultivated, and glorified. The obsession with merging with the other feeds precisely on their inaccessibility.

DOI: 10.4324/9781003728764-25

Passion and Perversion

Love, in a way, situates itself between passion and perversion. Passion and perversion are, on one hand, two poles that help ground love, yet on the other, they represent two extremes from which love must be protected. Colleague Michel Thys engagingly and illuminatingly plays with these contrasts.[4] In perversion, the subject suspends the relationship. By inserting something – a 'prop' or fetish, for instance – between themselves and the other, the other is not recognised as a person or as truly Other, but is kept at a distance and merely used as an instrument for drive-based satisfaction. In passion, by contrast, the subject does not suspend the relationship but rather overshoots it. In perversion, anything is possible; passion is governed by the impossible. Passion is love for the obstacle, while the perverse subject refuses to let anything stand in their way. The perverse person is both screenwriter and director, seizing power and exerting full control. By contrast, the passionate subject is enslaved by or surrendered to their own desire. Perversion destroys the other as a person, whereas passion is more likely to be destructive for the subject themselves.

Ordinary infatuation is delightful. One's mood is lifted, the world smiles back, and new possibilities bloom. But in passion, infatuation turns malignant. It hollows us out, narrows our gaze, and shrinks the world. It brings impoverishment rather than enrichment. What is at play is an absolute and unconditional attachment, in which we are seized by the ungraspable. This is the paradox of passion: we choose it, yet we have no choice at all. We feel compelled, claimed by it, passively subjected to its grip. The love-object is like the sun: it radiates a blistering heat and exerts immense suction and gravitational pull. It is an imperial *Roi/Reine Soleil.*

When attachment becomes unconditional, we inevitably draw close to the Thing.[5] The Thing may appear veiled, for instance, as an alluring and exceptional (love-)object. The lover is then led by a pure, nearly heroic desire for a beloved who comes to occupy the place of this Thing. In such a state, the lover becomes capable of anything and is beside themselves. They are bound to an intrinsic value, possessing the aesthetic and ethical qualities of the sovereign subject, and moving beyond the circuit of narcissism and self-interest. Independent of others, unbound by God or commandment, their desire is tethered to something that transcends judgments or advantages. They move in the direction of what lies *beyond.* Perhaps Nietzsche would call them someone with a swollen, clenched will[6] – someone who truly wills something or who desires something true: the Real Thing.

The Thing

But alas, when we are delivered to the horrifying nakedness of the Thing, the consequences can be devastating. David Lynch is one of those who vividly capture such horror on screen. The opening words of *Lost Highway* are heard through an intercom: 'Dick Laurent is dead.'[7] What follows are endless minutes in which the camera slowly and meticulously – yet with a faint sfumato quality – scans the interior of a house. It is as if one were descending a staircase in the dark, misplacing every step. The eye searches and searches, but there is nothing to see. Or rather, there is a nothingness that becomes the very site of an unbearable threat, as captured on film. The space becomes a vortex of illusion, drawing the viewer towards the Thing.

The intoxicating force of passion or rapture leads to an egoless enjoyment or a subjectless desire that teeters on the brink of self-destruction. It produces a transgressive pleasure in which the ego is no longer concerned with itself or guided by consequences. The subject, instead, proceeds untroubled, unrestrained, and unwaveringly towards its aim. It does not look back, is absorbed in its pursuit, blinded by its drive, outside itself (in XTC), and in full overdrive. The drive has become flesh.

But what exactly is this ego-less enjoyment and subject-less desire? They are nothing other than the energetic pleasure linked to the drive – a drive that has seized the reins and left the desiring subject behind. In this motion, the ego vanishes, and Being takes over. Slavoj Žižek describes this jouissance as the very place of *Dasein*.[8] And desire, he asserts, is a defence against that jouissance.

In the film *Body Heat*, William Hurt's character Ned Racine repeatedly circles the house of Kathleen Turner's Matty Walker.[9] She seems acutely aware of his presence and radiates nothing but seduction: embodied receptivity, active passivity. The heat hangs over the scene like a bell jar, and only occasionally do small bells chime in the wind. They function like a curtain – both veiling and revealing the Thing – an obstacle and a springboard all at once. When Ned Racine crosses the threshold, an excess of pleasure awaits him, but so does the threat of an inevitable and fatal conclusion.

Or consider *Romeo and Juliet*, the eponymous play by Shakespeare. Through their passion, they evolve into sovereign, mature individuals within days.[10] At the start of the play, Romeo is portrayed as a youth in the throes of puppy love. His affection for Rosaline feels unreal, lacking substance. He is not in love with Rosaline, but with love itself. Then comes the shock: his encounter with Juliet. Upon discovering that they belong to mutually hostile families, both are inflamed with a fiery passion. It is reminiscent of Jack and Rose in the film *Titanic*: the ship's sinking appears to be the obstacle to their love, but in reality, it is its necessary precondition.[11] The Schokker brothers thus argue that passion is only possible aboard a sinking ship.[12]

Likewise, the family feud is essential for Romeo to experience genuine passion – one that seizes him entirely, body and soul, and propels him beyond the threshold of maturity, away from his parental environment. Juliet, too, demonstrates acts of great inner strength for a 14-year-old: she inwardly breaks with her parents, separates from her nurse, and retreats into herself with an unwavering resolve to reach the utmost limit. Their mutual passion, their ecstasy, and their transgression mark for both a transition from paradisiacal childhood to responsible adulthood. But it cannot – must not – be. Their individuation fails. These adolescents do not succeed in finding a symbolic solution, a symptom to contain their passion. They remain as the two royal children separated by water too deep. Their passion short-circuits language, causing them to drown in the cool lakes of death. All passionate lovers thus become, to varying degrees, outlaws – like Bonnie and Clyde in the eponymous film,[13] or Lula and Sailor in *Wild at Heart*, again by David Lynch.[14] In the blindness of infatuation, as Freud already observed, one becomes a criminal without remorse.[15]

Tightrope

Eroticism is, in many respects, a balancing act on a tightrope. In his *Eleven Minutes*, Paulo Coelho aptly describes eroticism as the art of mastering the loss of control.[16] Desire and drive relate to one another like beauty to the beast, the known to the unknown. Desire honours the sign that reads: 'No Entry.' The desiring subject stops short of the deadly realm of jouissance. In doing so, the subject sustains the gap with the Thing, even within the most extreme relation. Drive, on the other hand, proceeds to completion with unyielding persistence. It plunges (self-)destructively into the Thing. It is, as Louis-Ferdinand Céline put it, a *Voyage au Bout de la Nuit* – a journey to the end of the night.[17]

In this context, we may distinguish between two forms of enjoyment: Dionysian and Apollonian, tension-increasing and tension-reducing.[18] Dionysian enjoyment is unlimited and symbiotic. This enjoyment lies beyond the pleasure principle, beyond language and signifier, beyond the phallus, and beyond gender differences. It is immediate enjoyment. This enjoyment signifies the death of the subject as subject. The subject disappears from the register of language and signifier. There is a free flow of energy according to a primary process. The enjoyment is total, merging and increasing tension, whereby the ego and subject disappear into the Other. They are incorporated, absorbed.

On the other hand, there is Apollonian enjoyment. It is phallic enjoyment or the lust that Freud usually talks about. Lacan also calls this '*la jouissance de l'idiot*,' the enjoyment of the idiot.[19] This lust offers a limited but safe enjoyment, in which the ego and subject continue to exist. This lust is partial, leads to separation and to a reduction in tension ('*la petite mort*') through orgasm, which brings an unwanted and abrupt end to the ecstatic, out-of-oneself state of enjoyment. Aristophanes' two-backed beast falls apart, and the lovers can say, 'I'm coming, I'm coming!' By climaxing, they also return as an I and as a subject. The loss of this temporary and illusory union makes every animal sad after the sexual act: '*Omne animal post coïtum triste.*'

Freud discussed the tension between tenderness and sensuality that complicates our love life in several texts. He consistently argues that humans do not easily integrate these two aspirations.[20] He considers this to be a consequence of our long-term dependence, the incest taboo, and the two (separated by a latency period) stages of our sexuality. He compared the difficulty to digging a tunnel, thereby indicating how delicate it is to align the two sides precisely. We find this idea again in the character of Thomas, the surgeon in Milan Kundera's *The Unbearable*

Lightness of Being.[21] According to Thomas, the protagonist, men experience two distinct passions. For him, love manifests itself not so much in the desire for copulation (a desire directed towards an infinite number of women) but in the desire for shared sleep (which can only be satisfied by a single, irreplaceable woman).

The split between *eros* and *thanatos*, or between the life drive and the death drive – which we have described through their distinct modes of enjoyment – introduces an additional complication into the experience of love.[22] It is a conflict that troubles human sexuality from within. We long for that which simultaneously terrifies us the most. Fusion with the Other inevitably carries the risk of losing ourselves.

Beyond the pleasure principle, a 'Good' begins to emerge – but it is a forbidden good: the Thing. It is towards this Thing that we orient ourselves, and it is this Thing that imposes the law. When Carmen sings in Bizet's opera, '*L'amour est un oiseau rebelle qui n'a jamais, jamais connu de loi*' ('Love is a rebellious bird that has never, ever known a law'), she is gravely mistaken. There exists, on the contrary, a primordial law to which love absolutely does submit – the law of the Thing. It is the law of caprice, a law that is, in a cruel and merciless – both for ourselves and for others. To follow this law is to reset the self in an act, as Jacques Lacan calls it.[23] By this, he means a symbolic, subjectivising act that structurally and irreversibly alters our relationships – including our relationship with our own unconscious.

This is one of the scandals – or rather, scandalous deeds – of psychoanalysis. Up until the Second World War, it was by far the dominant force in mental health care. In the words of Bruno Bettelheim, 'Just as the curing of bodily illnesses was that of medicine.'[24] Though temporarily eclipsed by the rise of psychopharmaceuticals and symptom-focused treatments like behaviour therapy, psychoanalysis has made a comeback in this millennium within the scientific world. In its more protocolled forms (such as Mentalisation-Based Treatment, Transference-Focused Psychotherapy, and Dynamic Interpersonal Psychotherapy), it has been included, for example, in the *Practice Guidelines* of the *American Psychiatric Association*.[25] Nevertheless, its ideas continue to be vilified — not only for their sexual content, but more fundamentally for their subversive potential.[26]

Heroes

To paraphrase André Breton, psychoanalysis forces the bourgeoisie to gaze into the abyss of nothingness. It certainly offers no guarantee for the establishment – or for what Lucebert, in his poem *9000 Jackals Swim to Boston*, called '*the Borobudur of the bourgeoisie*.'[27] Again and again, it approaches the Thing – a foreign body that disrupts the social order. It is a perilous proximity, one that requires hazardous decisions. These decisions can no longer rely solely on the imaginary of ideals or the symbolic order of norms and prohibitions, but must also reckon with the Real Thing. This can result in choices that may be deemed criminal or virtuous, worthy of admiration or of dread. They press against a boundary that life can only ever cross fleetingly.

In making an absolute choice, in performing an authentic act, the subject invariably experiences themselves as strange – even unintelligible – to themselves. And yet they assume full responsibility for that choice and accept it as something which, however foreign, defines their very being.

This notion may be further clarified through Lacan's reflections on the scoundrel, the ordinary man, and the hero.[28] The scoundrel is someone without a Superego, without conscience. Naturally, he is incapable of ethical action. The ordinary man is moral, even if he often thinks himself a scoundrel – or a narcissist, or a sex addict, and so on. Sometimes he seeks therapy for this. But when the ordinary man commits to his Thing, he takes on the position of the hero. From the perspectives of society and the superego, the hero is immoral. Yet he is ethical because he performs an authentic act. He may break the law, but he does not do so for personal gain, as the scoundrel does – he does it because he refuses to betray his desire. As David Bowie sings: *We can be heroes*. Though he adds, in the same breath: *Just for one day*. Anyone can play the hero, of course. But true heroism is reserved for a rare few – and it is, by necessity, short-lived.

Notes

1 De Rougemont, D. (1949). *Liefde en avondland*. Amsterdam: Uitgeversmaatschappij Holland.
2 Sartre, J. P. (1943/1976). *L'être et le néant*. Paris: Gallimard.
3 De Dijn, H. (Red.) (1999). *De uitgelezen Spinoza*. Amsterdam: Boom.
4 Thys, M. (2002). Liefde tussen perversie en passie? In M. Thys & M. Kinet (Red.), *Liefdesverklaringen. Over perversie, liefde en passie* (p. 9–21). Leuven-Leusden: Acco.
5 Moyaert, P. (1991). Fenomenologie van de eros. In H. Bleijendaal, J. Goud & E. Van Hove (Red.), *Emanuel Levinas over psyche, kunst en moraal* (pp. 33–45). Baarn: Ambo.
6 Nietzsche, F. (1901/2002). *De wil tot macht* (vert. P. H. van Rooden). Amsterdam: De Arbeiderspers, 2002 fragment 1067.
7 Lynch, D. (Director). (1997). *Lost highway* [Film]. October Films.
8 Žižek, S. (1992). *Enjoy your symptom*! London/New York: Routledge.
9 Kasdan, L. (Director). (1981). *Body heat* [Film]. Warner Bros.
10 Shakespeare, W. (1609/2023). *Romeo and Juliet* (G. B. Evans, Ed.; H. Lees-Jeffries, Int.). London: Cambridge University Press.
11 Cameron, J. (Director). (1997). *Titanic* [Film]. Paramount Pictures; 20th Century Fox.
12 Schokker, J. & Schokker, T. (2000). *Extimiteit. Jacques Lacans terugkeer naar Freud*. Amsterdam: Boom.
13 Penn, A. (Director). (1967). *Bonnie and Clyde* [Film]. Warner Bros.-Seven Arts.
14 Lynch, D. (Director). (1990). *Wild at heart* [Film]. PolyGram Filmed Entertainment.
15 Freud, S. (1914/2006). *Ter introductie van het narcisme*. In W. Oranje (Red. & Vert.), *Werken 6: Psychoanalytische theorie 1* (pp. 329–355). Amsterdam: Boom.
16 Coelho, P. (2003). *Elf minuten*. Amsterdam: Arbeiderspers.
17 Céline, L.-F. (1932/2020). *Voyage au bout de la nuit* (Édition anniversaire). Paris: Gallimard.
18 Paglia, C. (1992). *Het seksuele masker*. Amsterdam: Prometheus.
19 Lacan, J. (1973–1974/1975). *Le Séminaire Livre XX. Encore*. Texte établi par J. A. Miller. Paris: Du Seuil.

20 Freud, S. (1912). *Bijdragen tot de psychologie van het liefdeleven II: Over de meest verbreide vernedering in het liefdeleven. K.B.2. Sigmund Freud Nederlandse Editie* (pp. 183–198). Amsterdam/Meppel: Boom.
21 Kundera, M. (1985). *De ondraaglijke lichtheid van het bestaan.* Amsterdam: Ambo.
22 Freud, S. (1920). *Aan gene zijde van het lustprincipe.* P.T.1. Sigmund Freud Nederlandse Editie (pp. 95–163). Amsterdam/Meppel: Boom.
23 Lacan, J. (1967–1968/2016). *Le Séminaire, Livre XV: L'acte psychanalytique* (J.-A. Miller, Éd.). Paris: Seuil.
24 Bettelheim, B. (1983). *Freud and man's soul.* London: Hogarth Press.
25 American Psychiatric Association. (2010). *Practice guideline for the treatment of patients with borderline personality disorder.* Washington, DC: American Psychiatric Association Publishing.
26 Fisher, S. (2023). *The subversive edge of psychoanalysis.* London/New York: Routledge.
27 Lucebert. (1974). *Verzamelde Gedichten.* Amsterdam: Bezige Bij.
28 Schokker, J., & Schokker, T. (2000). *Extimiteit. Jacques Lacans terugkeer naar Freud.* Amsterdam: Boom.

Panoramic Intermezzo III

Where love becomes truly serious, the other no longer appears as a dream but as a symptom.

In this third movement, love becomes clinically visible: in transference, in therapy, in the couple, in generations, in hatred, perversion and passion.

The enchantment of the beginning gives way to the stubbornness of repetition.

Love proves not to be a purely chosen state but a fate: one loves where one is wounded, one repeats what one did not understand, one attaches oneself to what hurts because it is familiar.

The therapeutic space reveals that love does not heal through harmony, but through confrontation with what does not dissolve.

The beloved carries the symptom, the relationship becomes a stage upon which the unconscious performs itself.

What one reproaches in the other often belongs to one's own history.

Thus, love does not teach us how to become happy, but how to learn to endure.

Here love loses its innocence but gains in truth.

It becomes an adult when it acknowledges its fractures.

DOI: 10.4324/9781003728764-26

A Radiography of Seduction

Confiteor

I've been someone I never was,
Held up a mirror—then just glass.
I cheated, lied, played the game,
Used the Joker, took the fame.
What I knew, I chose to lose,
To dodge the shame of being true.
I borrowed words I didn't earn:
Passion, Mayakovsky, Zen—I let them burn.
I made you dance on sparks I spoke,
Blinded you with love I only wore like smoke.
So tear my feelings like old threadbare clothes,
So I can sleep—no guilt, no echoes.
Now that day fades out and night draws in,
I want to drop the act I've held within.

With these occasional verses, we introduce Vicomte de Valmont, the unrivalled grandmaster of seduction from *Les Liaisons Dangereuses* by Choderlos de Laclos.[1] His *confiteor* is, of course, pure fabrication, for the diabolical delight and power-lust that he and La Marquise de Merteuil derive from the ruin of unsuspecting innocents is far beyond remorse. One must admit that in their aristocratic pastime, they seem barely aware of any wrongdoing. Their victims are mere marionettes dancing to their exquisitely orchestrated tunes. In truth, both protagonists are primarily attempting to amuse, impress, and seduce one another.

In this timeless epistolary novel, seduction appears in an exaggerated, almost inhuman form. Beneath its hypercivilised and aristocratic façade, it defies law and convention, crosses boundaries, and thrives on the arts of flattery, charm, and intrigue. It convinces, surprises, unravels, paralyses. It suggests emotion rather than expressing it, all within an endless spectacle brimming with ambiguity and ulterior motives. Its victims are as innocent as children. We know what the decadents

DOI: 10.4324/9781003728764-27

thought of nature: too green and poorly lit. The opinion of these erotic predators about their prey runs along the same lines. Modesty does not inspire reverence but serves as an irresistible perfume of lust. Baudelaire aptly remarked that this novel burns as only ice can burn.[2]

Pure Animals

In contrast, the animal kingdom operates with purity and simplicity. Everything is preordained within the conglomerate of genes we call instinct. Sex and reproduction unfold according to a pre-programmed mechanism. In nature, it is not the females but the males who are the beauties. Phallic symbols such as tails, plumage, and ornamental displays govern courtship and mating rituals, which are further characterised by attraction and repulsion, and by distance and proximity. The alpha male earns his status through intrasexual selection – by battling rivals or by demonstrating his worth in other ways. There is also intersexual selection, where the alpha male outshines others by being a master of seduction. The sex difference is further marked by the passive/active opposition. The female carries large reproductive cells or macrogametes, motionless centres around which the more active and mobile male microgametes gravitate. The *survival of the fittest* begins with these merciless spermatozoa, engaged in fierce competition from the outset, each with one goal: to achieve fertilisation.

Similar (role) patterns can be observed among the *hominids*. Yet they are inevitably denatured and polymorphously perverted by the intrusion of language: a point to which we shall return. In human affairs, it is typically the female who is considered the fairest. She exhibits herself in polyandrous fashion within the amphitheatre populated by male voyeurs. By baring her neck, she simulates submission. The gaze is raised, the head turned slightly and inclined. In this way, she deftly manipulates the size of her eyes. And of course, the lips remain slightly parted in moist anticipation. As Freud notes in relation to the timing of interpretation, '*Le lion ne saute qu'une fois*' (the lion pounces only once).[3] And what better bait, what greater explosive potential, than a helpless or otherwise distressed female? Often, this unfolds more covertly, more enigmatically. A glance can say everything, yet it can always be denied. And besides, isn't eye contact invisible to third parties?

Let us, in passing, note a less orthodox interpretation of the Fall, one that centres precisely around the serpent of seduction. Because we could not resist this temptation, we were cast out of Paradise as punishment. Eve, the leading lady, functions as *prima peccatrix* (the original sinner), seducing Adam with her apple. And one needn't be a Flemish Primitivist to see in that apple not the maternal breast but the erotic breast, which is thus prohibited by the Father. To bite into it is the erotic reverse of the psychoanalytic original sin. It is the sensual counterpart to the primal murder of the father, which, according to Freud's *Totem and Taboo*, installs law, order, and guilt.

Anthropological Difference

Traditionally, the so-called 'anthropological difference', what separates us from our animal kin, is attributed to art, science, and religion. In humans, sexual signals and symbols are not straightforward signs. It is not the Porsche, but the French two-horsepower car (Citroën's *deux-chevaux*) that is considered the sexiest in some circles. A shabby vest may ignite more sparks than an Armani tie, and a demure maiden may well lose out to a cat in boots. In this regard, human signals and symbols are not mere signs, but signifiers. Their unstable meanings are determined by both the diachronic and synchronic contexts in which they appear. Just as the meaning of dream elements only emerges in relation to the transference dynamic, life history, and the dreamer's free associations. Psychoanalysis teaches us that there is no encyclopaedia of symbols in which every meaning can be conveniently found under alphabetical headings.

Malicious and loving seduction differ in that the former is calculated and conscious, while the latter is spontaneous and unconscious. Yet both operate according to the same principles and techniques. It is a comedy of the mind, where the ends justify the means and where sincere lies and false promises wrestle for dominance. The motto is well known: *All is fair in love and war*. The bottom line is that the man must be stroked in his actions and/or achievements: a compliment that flatters his Guinness Book of Records hysteria (Paul Verhaeghe) to be/have the longest, the biggest, the strongest.[4] The woman, in turn, must be stroked in whatever (minor) detail of her physical appearance – eyes, voice, hands – that gives her the sense of being a treasure. In psychoanalytic terms, these are narcissistic gratifications exchanged in veiled and/or opaque ways.

In humans, seduction unfolds not only in the imaginary realm but also in the symbolic register of language. At times, it is even less a matter of the right or most beautiful words than of their resonance. Courtly love and lyric poetry are, according to De Rougemont in *L'Amour et l'Occident*, constitutive of romantic love.[5] The troubadour's song seeks both to install and to overcome distance through a never-ending flow of sublimation. Words not only describe feelings but evoke them. The necessary rhetorical component renders all eroticism essentially fictive. In the game of seduction, what is said rarely coincides with what is meant. The most important element of any conversation is the subtext. The fundamental question is not 'Who am I?' but rather 'Who or what am I for the Other?' And above all: 'Does the Other desire me?' How should I be – how must I become – to arouse the Other's desire?

Phallic Peekaboo

Here, we must introduce the phallus as understood in Lacanian terms. In Freud and in everyday language, the phallus refers to a (male) anatomical organ that, from birth, marks sexual difference. For Lacan, the phallus is a signifier; one that is, as it were, provided to us by nature. The phallus signifies both desire and lack. In an epigrammatic formulation, Paul Verhaeghe describes the phallus as that which we can never possess or be enough of, a compensation for the lack in the Other.[6] In this capacity, it plays a pivotal role in seduction. Both parties engage in a game of peek-a-boo with this phallus. They present themselves as the answer to each other's lack, only to undermine that *semblant*/semblance. Both desire to be desired, yet both fear being reduced to a passive object of the Other's desire. According to Lacan, anxiety is primarily tied to the encounter with the Real: the Thing-in-itself, drive, and trauma. But also to the encounter with the Other's desire. As his famous analogy has it: what if I am caught *in flagrante delicto* as that which the praying mantis lacks, and the erotic play becomes a nightmare in which I vanish between her jaws?

Seduction Theories

Freud initially developed a trauma (or seduction) theory to explain the aetiology of neuroses. In this theory, the child is understood as the passive recipient of sexual advances from adults. These transgressions are enigmatic, unintegrated, and persist as foreign bodies within the psyche. Only later – post-puberty – do they acquire their pathogenic and traumatic charge retroactively. The patient then begins to suffer from their memories. Upon abandoning his *Neurotica*, Freud shifted his emphasis from external to psychic reality, and from memory to fantasy, though without denying the potential reality of trauma.[7] Yet seduction also exists in a broader, more structural sense. Not as accidental trauma, but as a universal condition. Inevitably, there arises a confusion of tongues between the child's playful, tender language and the adult's language of sexual passion. Following analysts like Sándor Ferenczi and Jean Laplanche, Julia Kristeva writes in the opening of *Histoires d'Amour* about the irreducibly traumatic nature of human sexuality.[8]

Within the (care-)giving nursing mother resides a darker, feminine side – one that is enigmatic and threatening. Bracha Ettinger refers to her as the *femme fatale Autre Mère*.[9] Her *Gestalt* can be recognised in mythical figures such as harpies, sirens, and gorgons, as well as in Semiramis, Helen of Troy, or Cleopatra. But also in characters like *La Traviata*, Zola's *Nana*, or Wedekind's *Lulu*. In any case, seduction is an intrinsic part of maternal care in its fleshy, embodied dimension. Very early in childhood, a tango begins, for the child too will attempt to seduce. This may take the form of imitation or mimicry, a response to maternal seduction. But the child might also seduce in order to affirm its own value or test the solidity of the Other. These seductive gestures may stem from a lack of self-confidence, from feeling unloved or abandoned, or from a drive born of despair.

Is not the latter Don Juan – a man who seeks to conquer yet another ('*mille e tre*') maternal woman – at heart a poor wretch? And is the father of the dishonoured Donna Anna (alias the *Commendatore*), who finally comes knocking, not in truth the absent father arriving far too late? From a Lacanian point of view, the father serves not only to forbid the mother to the child, but also to forbid the child from the mother. Beyond his prohibitive role, he thus fulfils a protective function that is at least as vital for the child's free development.

Spleen Pour Rire

Not all women hail from Venus, and many are poor map-readers. The reality of the consulting room makes clear that the evolutionary and neurobiological speculations underpinning such popular tropes bear little resemblance to what truly unfolds between human ears. For animals, sex and reproduction are instinctively programmed needs. Within the species, mating proceeds in a straight line from courtship to copulation. Not so for humans, who mirror their sexual relations on those of the Other (films, books, media, neighbours, parents…) and/or invent their own. Not so for humans, whose erotic life is shaped not only by biological instinct, but also – and above all – by (symbolic) complexes. Not so for humans, who may engage in sex with animals, plants, or corpses; who kiss, lick, or suck; who, dressed in latex or thongs, armed with strawberries or riding crops, pursue pleasure until death (sometimes even literally, as in cases of erotic asphyxiation). Not so for humans, whose sexuality is thus denatured, fundamentally maladapted, a mysterious, always particular and perverse cocktail of love and pornography.

The contemporary myth is that of the couple, sweating together with varying success, climaxing in unison. Yet beyond the anatomical mismatch lies the chasm of irreconcilable sexual difference. The man falls short, the woman wants more. In the masquerade of seduction, man and woman appear to one another as prince and *Ma Dame*. But more princes turn into frogs than frogs who become princes. And what lies hidden beneath the (chastity) belt of the lady? A crude and sexist joke has it that the ideal woman is one metre tall, has thick lips, and a flat head on which to rest your pint. In the best-case scenario, love in this view veils a dark duet between a frog and a pleasure object.

In any case, language and culture disrupt natural immediacy. The result is the *condition humaine*. In the words of Flemish modernist poet Paul Van Ostaijen, it can sometimes be a '*spleen pour rire*': a spleen (whether or not) to laugh about.[10]

Notes

1 De Laclos, C. (1782/2003). *Les liaisons dangereuses*. Paris: Gallimard Folio.
2 Baudelaire, C. (1866/1986). *Mon coeur mis à nu*. Paris: Gallimard Folio.
3 Freud, S. (1937/2006). De eindige en de oneindige analyse. In *Freud Werken* (Vol. 10, pp. 270–305). Amsterdam: Boom.
4 Verhaeghe, P. (1998). *Liefde in tijden van eenzaamheid*. Leuven: Acco.
5 De Rougemont, D. (1949). *Liefde en avondland*. Amsterdam: Uitgeversmaatschappij Holland.
6 Verhaeghe, P. (2002). *Over normaliteit en andere afwijkingen*. Leuven/Leusden: Acco.
7 Freud, S. (1905). *Drie verhandelingen over de theorie van de seksualiteit*. K.B.**1**. Sigmund Freud Nederlandse Editie (pp. 49–177). Amsterdam/Meppel: Boom.
8 Kristeva, J. (1985). *Histoires d'amour*. Paris: Gall.
9 Ettinger, B. (2006). *The matrixial borderspace. Essays by Bracha Ettinger*. Minneapolis: University of Minnesota Press.
10 Van Ostaijen, P. (1926/1996). Spleen pour rire. In *Verzamelde gedichten*. Amsterdam: Bert Bakker.

25

The Sweetest Lust

Contraception

Undoubtedly, the pill introduced in 1961 ranks among the most important inventions of the twentieth century. Of course, the method of *coitus interruptus* already had a long-standing tradition, but it was notoriously unreliable and hardly any fun. In 1844, the Goodyear company (better known for its tyres) brought a rubber condom to market. It was tough, awkward to use, and hardly an overwhelming success. Then came the Ogino-Knaus temperature method, which aimed to anticipate ovulation and fertility. This contraceptive method soon received the blessing of Pope Pius XII from Vatican City, and the mercury thermometer gained a permanent place alongside the crucifix in many bedrooms.

It was oral contraceptives that truly ushered in sexual liberation. As the pop lyric goes: 'I put you on a pedestal, you put me on the pill.' And that, supposedly, settled the matter. Sexuality could now finally be severed from reproduction, and marital duty evolved into what I once read scrawled on the wall of a public loo: 'Only when the spouses have truly enjoyed, has the couple truly coupled.' In other words, it is no longer the sexual act itself but (multi-)orgasmic enjoyment that has become a duty. Paul Verhaeghe frequently refers to the myth of the Masters and Johnson couple, who frantically strive to climax simultaneously.[1] With groans, lovers try to convince each other of their ecstatic rapture, and with panting, they send the message that they are too passionate to think. The precise location of the clitoris has since become the world's most important entrance exam. And since its 'discovery' in 1950 by Ernst Gräfenberg, the G-spot – credited in sexological literature since 1981 with triggering the cherry on the cake of female ejaculation – has attracted as many curious seekers as the Loch Ness Monster once did.

Salonfähig

Everyone knows the famous drawing of Freud in which his forehead resembles a female nude. Undeniably, his writings brought sexuality into public discourse, if not quite making it *salonfähig*, then at least discussable. Many still regard him

DOI: 10.4324/9781003728764-28

as the prophet of sexual liberation, though that title might more rightly belong to Wilhelm Reich. Freud himself certainly did not consider it a laughing matter to extract the secrets of infantile sexuality from reluctant adults. He often lamented that discussions of his theories were met not with arguments but with sentiment.[2] Still, he was unequivocal: 'Every human being contains repressed perverse elements, just as every organic molecule contains carbon, oxygen, hydrogen, and nitrogen – albeit in differing proportions.'[3] In his defence, he claimed merely to have brought the sexual drives to attention, just as the chemist reduces all compounds to their chemical affinities. Laconically, Freud added that the chemist does not deny the existence of other forces, such as gravity, but leaves their analysis to others, for example, the physicist.

Freud initially approached love through the lens of infantile sexuality, which he mapped in 1905 in connection with various perversions. The relationship with the mother's breast – as a source of nourishment, warmth, and safety – serves, according to Freud, as the prototype of all future love relations. Finding a love 'object' is essentially a re-finding of this early prototype. We are drawn to maternal features in the beloved: her smile, gaze, voice, or gestures. During the latency period of early school years, cognitive development takes centre stage, and due to incestuous connotations, the sexual current of this early love is repressed, leaving only the tender stream consciously active. In adolescence, the sexual current is typically detached from its original incestuous object and redirected towards a non-incestuous one. But this process is not without complications.

A major development in Freud's theory of love came with his introduction of narcissism.[4] It appears we seek to (re)find ourselves in the other. Unknowingly, we continue to search (also in the other, or what Lacan would call the *petit autre* or other-like-self) for something of ourselves. Our partner choice lies between two poles: the narcissistic, in which the other is chosen based on who/how I am, was, or wish to be; and the anaclitic, in which the other corresponds to the image of the nurturing mother or the protective father. In the latter, partner choice is based on self-preservative drives. Falling in love, in this light, is a disguised form of self-love, for the beloved becomes the (imaginary) projection of one's own Ideal Ego.

Love Psychology

Freud continued to make extensive contributions to the psychology of love. He described, for instance, several 'favourable' love conditions: the allure of a woman who is unavailable, already bound to a third party; the erotic appeal of a woman with a tainted reputation – the so-called 'whorish' woman; and all desires for tenderness, gratitude, and lust that, ultimately, are driven by the wish to become one's own father. He also addressed some of the most common sexual difficulties, especially those rooted in the split between tenderness and sensuality, between heavenly and earthly – animalistic – love. As Triggerfinger's song puts it: 'God has your head, the devil has your balls.'[5]

A phenomenon Freud identified as particularly widespread is the combination of devaluation of the sexual object and idealisation of the incestuous one.[6] This is the result of fixations on the mother, aunt, or sister – or, conversely, on the father, uncle, or brother. Such strong infantile fixations collide with the incest taboo, leading to the long period of sexual dormancy that characterises the latency phase in childhood. Freud thus suggests that sexual inhibition may be the rule rather than the exception. To be sexually free, one must have overcome both the reverence for – and idealisation of – the opposite sex. One must be able to use and be used by the other sexually. One must also have become familiar with incestuous representations and fantasies. We are all 'motherfuckers.'

Freud also observed that the intensity of erotic desire tends to decrease as its satisfaction becomes more easily attainable. In his words, an obstacle is needed to elevate the libido. He even suggests that humans may have invented conventions precisely in order to heighten pleasure. According to La Rochefoucauld, absence diminishes mediocre passion but intensifies great passion, just as wind extinguishes candles but kindles fire.[7]

One More Drink

How idyllic and harmonious is the relationship between the alcoholic and his favourite drink: an object of lifelong loyalty, even unto death. Something in the sexual drive, by contrast, seems inherently at odds with complete satisfaction. Freud offers two reasons for this. First, the choice of a love object occurs in two stages, separated by the incest barrier. Second, the ultimate sexual object is no longer the original one, but a substitute. The instability of object choice and the hunger for new stimuli result in a never-ending series of replacements. As Blaise Pascal put it, desire feeds on change.[8] In *The Beautiful and the Damned*, F. Scott Fitzgerald compares the desired to something that briefly glimmers in a shaft of sunlight, only to be inescapably overtaken by shadow and lose its brilliance moments later.[9]

Reconciling the claims of the drive with the demands of civilisation was, for Freud, a *mission impossible*. Renunciation, suffering, and (ultimately) the looming extinction of the human species seemed to him inevitable. On the other hand, this tormenting human condition also gives rise to sublimation, expressed in cultural achievements of varying magnificence. For if we were capable of complete satisfaction, why would we bother with anything else? What need would there be for 'progress?' 'Make love, not war' may sound like a sexy motto, but in practice it proves less simple to realise – even after the so-called sexual liberation.

Decline and Fall

Large-scale surveys show that sexual activity among young people today is declining rather than increasing, despite the omnipresence of sex in the media.[10] The so-called 'evaporation of sex' seems to have had a counterproductive effect.[11] Sex and sexuality must therefore be distinguished. Sex is a fleeting phenomenon, while sexuality encompasses the whole of one's personality. Realising its dimensions is a complex, lifelong endeavour that involves both body and mind, is simultaneously interpersonal and intrapsychic, and grants fantasy life a central role. Public 'pornification' has become detached from any psychosocial or sociocultural context. The pressure to perform increases, and desire buckles under it. As Iris Osswald-Rinner puts it, we are all both 'oversexed and underfucked.'[12]

Karl Kraus, polemicist and contemporary of Freud, provocatively argued that coitus is but an inadequate substitute for masturbation. Love, by contrast, is total. It involves a mutual orientation toward the other and their desire. The coupling of love and sexuality, then, is far from self-evident. The field of the drive is directed toward partial objects – mouth, breasts, penis, vagina, anus, etc. – and toward a pursuit of pleasure that threatens love from within. This pursuit is auto-erotic and polymorphous perverse. The repression of infantile sexuality is, for Freud, the principal explanation for all kinds of sexual inhibitions. The inevitable guilt that accompanies activities in the genital zone, and the inherently conflictual nature of such acts, more broadly explain the secrecy that perpetually cloaks the sexual relation. Couples desire to deny their guilt. By ignoring the gazes and stories of others, they short-circuit all envy and accusation. But in reverse, according to Otto Kernberg, it is precisely the renunciation of childhood sexual taboos that cements the emotional, cultural, and social life of the couple.[13]

Donald Meltzer distinguishes between infantile and mature polymorphous sexuality. The latter is discreet, modest, needs no display, and respects the privacy of one's own intimate experiences as well as those of the partner. It is not about power. In foreplay, early relationships and perverse elements are repeated – not repressed, but celebrated – and reinforce the shared intimacy.[14]

Enjoy!

Physical satisfaction, of course, is not the same as enjoyment. The former is mute organ-pleasure. Lacan called this phallic *jouissance*. Statistics about the number of conquests or orgasms point to a link with language – after all, the man must be able to tell (or count) them. This form of *jouissance* consolidates masculine self-esteem and is localised in specific erogenous zones. These are zones governed by the law and order of the Symbolic order. They were forbidden to the child, and are all the more exciting because of that prohibition.

Feminine or 'supplementary' *jouissance* exceeds these limits. It is characterised – regardless of chromosomes or anatomy – by a different form of enjoyment. Pleasure takes place as much between the ears as between the legs. It is a phantasmatic event and fundamentally symbolic–imaginary in nature. In sexual pleasure, the lack is only overcome in fantasy. Enjoyment becomes possible only insofar as what is forbidden by the law is realised in fantasy. The libertine who consciously seeks unbounded enjoyment will ultimately be disappointed – for *the Real Thing* is unpleasurable. It belongs to the desolate universe of the Marquis de Sade.

William Blake seems to consider sex to be the tree of nature on which we are hanged.[15] Reproduction and death are the red threads of the species.[16] Menstruation is a curse.[17] The first ejaculation is a pollution.[18] Upon Louis XIV's first nocturnal emission, the courtiers are said to have whispered: '*Le roi se meurt*' ('The king is dying').[19] Leonardo da Vinci found the sexual act revolting.[20] Baudelaire compared it to torture or a surgical operation ('*triste sensualité!*')[21] or, as Mallarmé sighed, '*La chair est triste, hélas*!'[22]

In sexuality, we lose ourselves, we lose the other, we lose ourselves in the other – and in otherness. We are both outside our body (*hors-corps*) and inside it (*en-corps*).[23] We leave ourselves through fantasy, even as our organs partake in pleasure. We imagine ourselves in seventh heaven, only to be reminded by sex of our grounding in flesh and the forces of gravity.

Notes

1 Verhaeghe, P. (1998). *Liefde in tijden van eenzaamheid.* Leuven: Acco.
2 Freud, S. (1905). *Drie verhandelingen over de theorie van de seksualiteit.* K.B.**1**. Sigmund Freud Nederlandse Editie (pp. 49–177). Amsterdam/Meppel: Boom.
3 Freud, S. (1905). *Drie verhandelingen over de theorie van de seksualiteit.* K.B.**1**. Sigmund Freud Nederlandse Editie (pp. 49–177). Amsterdam/Meppel: Boom.
4 Freud, S. (1914). *Ter introductie van het narcisme.* P.T. **1**. Sigmund Freud Nederlandse Editie (pp. 27–64). Amsterdam/Meppel: Boom.
5 Triggerfinger. (2010). *Tuxedo.* In All this dancin' around. Excelsior Recordings.
6 Freud, S. (1912). *Bijdragen tot de psychologie van het liefdeleven II: Over de meest verbreide vernedering in het liefdeleven.* K.B.**2.** Sigmund Freud Nederlandse Editie (pp. 183–198). Amsterdam/Meppel: Boom.
7 De La Rochefoucauld. (1665/2008). *Maximen – bespiegelingen over menselijk gedrag,* vert. Maarten van Buuren. Groningen: Historische Uitgeverij.
8 Pascal, P. (1664/2000). *Gedachten.* Amsterdam: Boom.
9 Fitzgerald, F. S. (1922/1995). *The beautiful and the damned.* New York: Scribner.
10 Podcast Sex in the Media, *Die Zeit* d.d. 25/09/2017.
11 Parin, P. (1986). Die Verflüchtigung des Sexuellen. *Diess. Subjekt im Widerspruch, S. 81–90.*
12 Osswald-Rinner, I. (2011). *Oversexed and underfucked: Über die gesellschaftliche Konstruktion der Lust.* Wiesbaden: VS Verlag für Sozialwissenschaften.
13 Kernberg, O. F. (1998). *Love relations: Normality and pathology.* New Haven-London: Yale University Press.
14 Meltzer, D. (1990). *Sexual states of mind.* Perthshire: Clunie Press.
15 Blake, W. (1790–1793/2008). *The marriage of heaven and hell* (M. A. Green, Ed.). Oxford: Oxford University Press.
16 Bluche, F. (1986/1990). *Louis XIV* (M. Prince, Trans.). New York,NY: Franklin Watts.
17 Bible, New Revised Standard Version. (1989). *Leviticus, 15,*19–30. National Council of Churches of Christ.
18 Douglas, M. (1966/2003). *Purity and danger: An analysis of concepts of pollution and taboo.* London/New York: Routledge.

19 Bluche, F. (1986/1990). *Louis XIV* (M. Prince, Trans.). New York, NY: Franklin Watts.
20 Leonardo da Vinci. (c. 1490–1519/2008). *The notebooks of Leonardo da Vinci* (I. MacCurdy, Ed.). Mineola, NY: Dover.
21 Baudelaire, C. (1866/1986). *Mon coeur mis à nu*. Paris: Gallimard Folio.
22 Mallarmé, S. (1865/1998). Brise marine. In B. Marchal (Ed.), *Poésies* (pp. 44–45). Paris: Gallimard.
23 Lacan, J. (1975). *Le Séminaire Livre XX. Encore*. Texte établi par J. A. Miller. Paris: Du Seuil.

26

Pornocracy

Pornocrates

In 1878, the Belgian artist Félicien Rops painted one of his most renowned works, titled *Pornocrates*, or *The Woman with the Pig*.[1] The woman is nude, wearing black stockings and gloves, and is blindfolded. She leads a pig with a golden tail on a leash. Her appearance immediately evokes associations with an S&M dominatrix. Since the episode in Homer's *Odyssey* involving Circe,[2] the symbolism of the pig is clear: it is the foolish man who dances to her tune. Or perhaps, conversely, the pig with its golden (!) tail has the upper hand, unconsciously or unwittingly pulling the strings. Maybe the tail refers less to Freud's penis than to Lacan's phallus. Are we, after Nietzsche's death of God, now left only to worship the Golden Calf? Has money become the ultimate currency of the phallus, giving us the illusion that, through it, the phallus can be bought? In any case, Rops' masterpiece is rich in sexual layering. The painting reflects not only ambivalence and ambiguity between active and passive, dominance and submission; it is also a vivid illustration of the fascination with and hatred towards the mysterious femme fatale, who, as Serge André suggests, is rooted in Freud's famous question to Marie Bonaparte: '*Was will das Weib*?'[3]

Pornography, of course, has existed in all eras, but with the advent of the internet, it is now available to everyone, free of charge, just a few clicks away – literally within reach. But what exactly constitutes the appeal of pornography? And why are predominantly men consuming it? To be clear: it is not that porn is only watched by men, but who has ever heard a man complain that women are watching *too much* porn?

Porn-Appeal

The appeal of pornography for men lies in the fact that it is *not* real, whereas for women, it is precisely its *realism* that makes it threatening. For men, pornography is a matter of fantasy (which they tend to distinguish clearly from reality), while for women, it is experienced in terms of reality. After all, aren't the men actually *doing things* to those women on screen?

DOI: 10.4324/9781003728764-29

On closer inspection, conscience is the great absentee in pornography. The 'stories' revolve around easy sexual expression – without inhibition, without shame. Conventional values are disrupted, and the viewer identifies not with interpersonal relationships but with a sexual act. There is no ambiguity or subtlety. The plot is a meaningless excuse for showcasing raw action. No fantasy is evoked around the inner life of the cardboard-cutout protagonists, which contributes to the sense of mechanisation. Polymorphously perverse, infantile impulses are aroused, dissociated from any form of tenderness. Sexuality, in the terms of Donald Winnicott, is ruthless, without concern, and developmentally prior to love.[4] For instance, the aggressive or sadistic components of pre-genital sexuality appear on full display, and there is a fetishistic degradation of the couple, reduced to a set of interchangeable (auxiliary) parts. The perverse decomposition of eroticism severs its link with aesthetic experience and the idealisation of passionate love.

The woman becomes nothing more than a sex object: complete with breast implants, vulvoplasty, and a perpetually moist vagina: a Valhalla for the helmet-haired, spear-wielding Achilles. He thrusts away, while she gazes into the camera with the cliché expression of eager arousal – nothing but a simulated display of subjectivity.

However crude (and seemingly contradictory) it may seem, sexuality in pornography is simultaneously stripped of its object-like quality. Tasteless and odourless, image and sound remove any possible horror of the Real from the experience. The imagery is moulded entirely to suit hallucinatory wish-fulfilments, where the masculine stands firm and unambiguous, and the feminine seems to harbour but one desire: *I'll be your fantasy*. In short, what is pornography if not the visual support of masturbatory fantasies? Porn is instantly accessible, delivers intense stimuli, and remains entirely under personal direction and control, without dependence on the Big Other. It is the safest sex of all.

WYSIWYG

Research confirms that pornography is less about sexual liberation than about repression. A study involving 299 university students asked whether they perceived their porn consumption as problematic.[5] Did it, for example, lead to an increase in intrusive sexual thoughts or difficulties in forming compatible relationships? Pornography appeared to serve primarily as a mechanism for regulating sexual thoughts and feelings, and correlated more with inhibition (for instance, due to moral or religious reasons) than with disinhibition. The availability of taboo sexual experiences online seems to function as a siren song to these more 'neurotic' students – one that no mast or wax plug can protect them from.

To some extent, pornography has now fully permeated popular culture, and many 'modern women' have, to varying degrees, identified with it. A recent cartoon showed the evolution of the female mons pubis over the decades. It shifted from a tropical swamp to a polished slit – from hidden depths and mysteries to the transparency of *what you see is what you get*. The jungle of Gustave Courbet's famous painting *L'Origine du Monde* has been replaced by barren landscapes. Everything is neat and tidy, ready-made for bite-sized, risk-free, and hygienically approved industrial and consumer use.

From a classical Freudian perspective, there is often a gap between the devoted love for the mother–virgin and the sexual desire directed at the 'whore' figure. Both pornography and prostitution represent forms of love that can be purchased, allowing the man to stray with relatively little risk (provided he exercises a degree of caution). Michael Bader adds an important dimension to this picture. According to him, pornographic images function as a counterweight to the experience of a sad or damaged mother.[6] For many men, the perception that the woman in their sexual fantasy is enjoying herself serves as proof that she is not being harmed. He may be 'ruthless,' yet it appears not to affect her negatively.

He is seemingly allowed to suck her nipples or clitoris, lick or bite her, pull her hair, spank her, or take her from behind – all without guilt. It seems to give her the greatest pleasure. In this way, he can let himself go completely and experience full sexual arousal with a clear conscience. She wants nothing more than to have her various body parts used at his will. Is this not the classic or ultimate excuse for every man? 'She wanted it herself!'

Sexual Difference

There is no shortage of clichés about women being from Venus and men from Mars. Men are said to use love to obtain sex, while women use sex to obtain love. Another one: women need a reason for sex, men only need a location. But there is little value in oversimplifying or demonising sexual difference. Sexual fantasies (even those staged in real life, on stage, on screen, or digitally, complete with fellow players and props) must primarily be understood as attempts to feel sufficiently safe to allow oneself to become sexually aroused and let go.

For the boy, separation from the mother is more complex than for the girl. He must not only detach from her, but also from his identification *with* her. Masculinity, then, becomes the denial or rejection of femininity.[7] Closeness, intimacy, and dependence are considered feminine and must therefore be repudiated. When the boy distances himself from his mother, guilt arises because the maternal bond is damaged. Confusion ensues – between dependence and emotional connection, between healthy sexual ruthlessness and damaging aggression. Discovering the sex of the mother-woman is, moreover, a terrifying revelation. It is the unimaginably Real: the wound from which I originate.

According to Bader, the hidden and inverted logic of male sexuality is not that men treat women too much as objects, but rather too little.[8] It is not that they are insufficiently concerned, but that they are overly so. Not that they are selfish, but that they feel guilty. Responsibility, concern, sensitivity, shame, or fear of rejection – all these inhibit the capacity for sexual arousal. Sexual fantasies and scenarios are thus inventions – sophisticated psychodynamic mechanisms devised to counteract anxiety and worry, and to overcome obstacles to pleasure. Sexual preferences, then, are nothing more than fantasies that can be acted out (with mutual consent). When these match or 'click,' they cement the couple's psychosexual and sociocultural bond.[9]

Fantasy

The analysis of sexual preferences or fantasies (like the dream) is a royal road to the unconscious. What seems like 'natural' sexual attraction or arousal turns out, upon closer examination, to be a highly elaborate complex of deep and intricate meanings. In those few nanoseconds or 'microdots' of sexual magnetism – or, by extension, love at first sight – a full unconscious psychological life is reflected.[10] Through careful analysis, they offer a key to discovering our *Ding*, or as we might put it: 'what makes our clock (I originally wrote *cock*) tick.'

All human sexuality is (as Joyce McDougall suggested with her alternative term for perversion) a personal invention: a form of 'neosexuality.'[11] When we examine each individual separately and listen to each subject in their own right, sexuality becomes a label that covers the most diverse meanings. Every sexual fantasy and preference harbours an underlying archaic meaning, concealed beneath an eroticised scenario that delicately combines numerous themes and psychodynamic functions. If one does not fixate on the sexual practice itself but considers the personality as a whole, sexuality reveals itself as only one manifestation of a complex psychic condition in which erotic, aggressive, narcissistic, and other concerns are at play.

Notes

1 Rops, F. (1878/2015). Pornocrates, *ou La Dame au cochon.* In M. Félicien Rops (Ed.), *Félicien Rops: Œuvres graphiques* (pp. xx–xx). Namur: Éditions du Musée Félicien Rops.
2 Homer. (1919/1995). *The Odyssey* (A. T. Murray & G. E. Dimock Jr., Trans.). Cambridge, MA: Harvard University Press. (Loeb Classical Library), 10.135–574.
3 André, S. (1986) *Que veut une femme*? Paris: Seuil.
4 Winnicott, D. W. (1945/1992). Primitive emotional development. In *Through paediatrics to psycho-analysis* (p. 154). London: Karnac.
5 Twohig, M. P., Crosby, J. M., & Cox, J. M. (2009). Viewing internet pornography: For whom is it problematic, how and why? *Sexual Addiction & Compulsivity*, *16*(4), 253–266.
6 Bader, M. (2009). *Male sexuality. Why women don't understand it... And men don't either*. Plymouth: Rowman & Littlefield.
7 Freud, S. (1937). *De eindige en de oneindige analyse*. K.B.**4.** Sigmund Freud Nederlandse Editie (p. 305). Amsterdam/Meppel: Boom.
8 Bader, M. (2003). *Arousal: The secret logic of sexual fantasies*. New York: St Martin's Griffin.
9 Kernberg, O. F. (1998). *Love relations: Normality and pathology*. New Haven-London: Yale University Press.
10 Stoller, R. M. (1986). *Sexual excitement. Dynamics of erotic life* (p. 165 e.v.). London/New York: Karnac.
11 McDougall, J. (1986). Identifications, neoneeds and neosexualities. *International Journal of Psycho-Analysis*, *67*, 19–33.

27

Contemporary Love?

Liberation vs Liberalisation

In the early twenty-first century, Western societies appeared to have reached an unprecedented degree of sexual liberation. Sexuality, once constrained by moral taboos and religious prohibitions, had entered a phase of normalisation and commodification. Casual sex, multiple relationships, and the proliferation of dating apps were celebrated as symbols of autonomy and freedom. The so-called *hookup culture* (the social climate in which sexual encounters occur without emotional attachment or commitment) became both an emblem of progress and a target of moral anxiety. Its emergence coincided with neoliberal ideals of self-management and consumption: bodies and desires became items to be selected, optimised, and exchanged in the marketplace of affect.[1] Yet, curiously, this culture of erotic abundance coincides with a measurable decline in sexual activity among young people. Journalistic and academic reports began to describe what was soon called the *sex recession*.[2] Surveys in the United States and other Western countries revealed that members of Generation Z (those born after 1995) were having significantly less sex than previous cohorts. The data showed not only a decrease in casual encounters but also in romantic relationships and partnered intimacy. Nearly a third of young men and a fifth of young women in their early twenties reported no sexual activity during the preceding year.[3]

This phenomenon confounded social expectations. For the first time in modern history, public concern was not about the excess of youth sexuality, but its apparent disappearance. Earlier generations had been accused of moral laxity (from the countercultural revolution of the 1960s to the AIDS-ridden fears of the 1980s), but now commentators spoke of a generation that was, in Tolentino's words, 'surrounded by a Vegas buffet of carnality and yet losing its appetite.'[4] What had once been condemned as excess was now mourned as absence.

Several explanatory frameworks have been proposed. Sociologist Jean Twenge suggested that the decline is part of a broader pattern of delayed adulthood among the iGen, including later initiation into dating, work, and independence.[5] Economic insecurity, extended education, and the omnipresence of digital entertainment may all contribute to a withdrawal from embodied social life. Fewer people form stable

DOI: 10.4324/9781003728764-30

couples, and those who do so later in life, resulting in a structural reduction of opportunities for sexual contact.[6]

Libidinal Economy

Sociologists have described this new landscape as one of eros without binding, or lust detached from love.[7] Psychoanalytically, such detachment marks a shift from object love (where the other is recognised as a subject of desire) to narcissistic satisfaction, in which the other functions merely as a screen for self-gratification.[8] The hookup culture, initially perceived as liberation from repression, might thus conceal a deeper form of alienation: the incapacity to encounter the other *as* other. It is precisely this paradox that fuels the fascination of contemporary commentators. The decline in sexual activity is not simply a demographic curiosity but a symptom of broader transformations in subjectivity and sociality. The so-called *post-sexual* condition of Generation Z mirrors the disembodiment of the digital age. The smartphone, as Tolentino notes, offers a permanent interface between fantasy and solitude: it allows for infinite simulations of desire while shielding the user from the risks of embodied intimacy.[9] Sex becomes both omnipresent and inaccessible: a spectacle without touch.

Historically, every sexual revolution has been followed by a reaction. The liberation of the 1960s gave rise to the moral backlash of the 1980s; the digital explosion of the 2010s now seems to culminate in a form of abstinence that is less moral than existential. Some conservative voices, such as the British journalist Louise Perry, interpret the sex recession as a welcome correction: a return to seriousness about sexuality, an acknowledgement of the dangers of promiscuity, and a defence of traditional bonds.[10] Perry's *The Case Against the Sexual Revolution* argues that the asymmetry between male and female desire, grounded in biological vulnerability, necessitates caution and restraint. For her, the risks of casual sex outweigh its benefits for women, who bear greater emotional and physical costs.

Progressive critics view such positions as reactionary. Feminist philosopher Katherine Angel countered that consent alone cannot guarantee mutuality, since consent may occur within structures of inequality and exploitation.[11] For Angel, the challenge is not to repress desire but to re-imagine sexual ethics beyond transactional models. In a similar vein, cultural journalist Carter Sherman described the sexual landscape of Generation Z as caught between opposing forces: conservative moralism and the libertarian excess of the internet.[12] In her account, young people oscillate between the poles of prohibition and overexposure, neither of which fosters genuine erotic connection.

The Lack of Excess

This tension has profound psychoanalytic implications. Where Freud identified the repression of sexuality as the price of civilisation,[13] contemporary culture exhibits the inverse: an excess of representation that paradoxically produces inhibition.

Desire, stripped of its mystery and distance, becomes inert. The 'pornographic unconscious,' as Han calls it, transforms erotic energy into visual data, measurable likes, and algorithmic feedback.[14] The Other is no longer a subject to be desired but an image to be consumed.

The sex recession is not simply about fewer sexual acts but about a reconfiguration of the libidinal economy itself. The sexual act (once a privileged site of encounter, risk, and transformation) has been displaced by the management of desire through screens. The erotic, in Audre Lorde's sense of a vital, creative force that resists domination, is replaced by a commodified simulation of pleasure.[15] As a result, the contemporary subject faces not repression but saturation, not prohibition but numbness.

The psychoanalytic reading thus invites a reversal of the usual lament: perhaps young people are not losing their appetite for sex but are defending themselves against an unbearable surplus of stimulation. In a world where desire is constantly solicited, withdrawal may function as a form of resistance. It is a refusal to participate in the relentless circulation of images and expectations. The sex recession, then, could be read not merely as a decline but as a symptom: a sign of psychic fatigue, a silent protest against the commodification of intimacy.

Technological Desire

If the first riddle of the sex recession lies in the coexistence of sexual abundance and erotic withdrawal, its second resides in the technological mediation of desire. Never before has sex been so visible, searchable, and apparently accessible. The smartphone, that pocket-sized prosthesis of subjectivity, now functions as both a stage and a filter for intimacy. Through dating apps and social media, desire becomes algorithmically organised: swipes, likes, and matches replace the contingencies of encounter. Technology promises connection while delivering control; it offers the fantasy of infinite choice while, in practice, producing unprecedented isolation.[16] Kate Julian's empirical portrait in *The Atlantic* revealed that digital mediation has profoundly altered not only how people meet, but how they imagine intimacy itself.[17] Online dating, far from accelerating sexual contact, often results in what she calls 'option paralysis.' Faced with endless potential partners, individuals struggle to choose, fearing that every match might preclude a better one. The paradox of abundance becomes the anxiety of selection. Psychological research has long shown that too many options reduce satisfaction and motivation: a dynamic amplified by the gamified design of dating apps. Swiping produces micro-doses of dopamine, rewarding the anticipation of connection more than connection itself.[18]

For many users, the result is not erotic liberation but exhaustion. Tinder's internal data indicate that the average user spends more than an hour per day on the app; however, only a fraction of matches translate into conversations, and even fewer into real encounters.[19] The sexual marketplace thus mirrors the neoliberal economy: hypercompetitive, self-branding, and ultimately lonely. The self must appear desirable yet self-sufficient, available yet autonomous. It is a tension that corrodes the very conditions of reciprocity.

Psychoanalysis offers a lens for understanding this dynamic. In Lacanian terms, digital platforms transform the *objet petit a*, the elusive cause of desire, into a series of images that promise satisfaction but deliver repetition. Desire, which thrives on absence and delay, becomes trapped in the circuitry of instant gratification. The screen becomes a mirror that reflects only the self's commodified version, rendering the other superfluous. The more one seeks the Other, the more one encounters only oneself.

Pornography

The omnipresence of pornography intensifies this structural impasse. Nearly three-quarters of young Americans have encountered online pornography by the age of eighteen, and many before adolescence.[20] The internet thus serves as a global school of the libido, shaping expectations and fantasies before embodied experience can intervene. The 'pornographic imagination' operates not as an addition to reality but as its replacement: it teaches that sex is a spectacle, that bodies are functions, and that pleasure can be achieved without the risk of reciprocity.[21] Pornography's ubiquity is not new, but its digital form is unprecedented in speed, quantity, and isolation. As Julian observed, masturbation and solitary arousal have surged in tandem with online availability. The 'sex for one' culture, as she terms it, is neither simply pathological nor harmless. It reflects a shift from relational to autoerotic modes of satisfaction. In Freud's vocabulary, libido has regressed from object-love to narcissistic investment[22]; in Winnicott's language, the potential space of play between self and other has collapsed into the closed circuit of self-stimulation.[23]

The consequences are not only behavioural but phenomenological. Many young adults report that their porn life and sex life are entirely disconnected. The digital body, infinitely malleable and devoid of resistance, contrasts sharply with the unpredictability of an actual partner. The more one consumes visual representations of sex, the more the real becomes unbearable – too slow, too ambiguous, too dependent on mutual attunement. Desire thus migrates from encounter to image, from intersubjective risk to solitary control. From a socio-economic perspective, pornography exemplifies what Han calls the 'achievement society' of transparency and performance.[24] Pleasure becomes a measurable productivity, a self-optimisation of arousal. The subject becomes both producer and consumer of its own excitation. The sex recession may not signal a lack of sexuality but its full integration into capitalist rationality. Desire is no longer repressed; it is managed.

Dating

The same ambivalence pervades the world of dating apps. Although initially associated with the liberation of sexual choice, apps like Tinder and Bumble increasingly function as mechanisms of self-surveillance. They encourage users to curate identities, measure attractiveness, and internalise rejection through data. The erotic is thus displaced from the body to the interface. As Tolentino remarks, the smartphone offers the illusion of endless availability while fostering a chronic fear of exposure.[25] To appear desirable is to risk humiliation; to protect oneself is to remain unseen. In this environment, intimacy becomes both desired and dreaded. The *hookup culture* (ostensibly about freedom) turns out to mask a profound anxiety about attachment. Psychodynamic clinicians have noted a rise in patients who express longing for connection but panic when confronted with vulnerability.[26] The digital screen offers safety without touch, conversation without silence, and fantasy without frustration. All the elements that, in psychoanalytic theory, sustain psychic growth are neutralised.

It is striking that, despite the proliferation of dating platforms, the rates of romantic coupling and marriage continue to decline.[27] Even those who use apps regularly describe them not as paths to relationships but as forms of entertainment, comparable to casual gaming or social scrolling. Julian cites young users who confess to downloading Tinder 'when bored,' enjoying the validation of being 'right-swiped' without any intention of meeting.[28] Desire becomes aesthetic rather than erotic; the libido circulates without aim, like capital without investment.

This process exemplifies what Marx described as *commodity fetishism*: social relations mediated by things.[29] In the digital economy of desire, the Other is both product and consumer. The subject becomes an entrepreneur of its own desirability, competing for attention in an image market. Illouz has argued that emotional life under late capitalism is organised around the logic of exchange: love becomes a rationalised investment, and disappointment a form of depreciation.[30] The sex recession, then, is not merely about the absence of sex but the collapse of erotic meaning under the weight of calculation.

Flatscreens

Some critics, like psychologist Philip Zimbardo (renowned for his Stanford Prison Experiment), have sought biological explanations, attributing diminished libido to dopamine habituation or 'porn-induced erectile dysfunction.'[31] While such hypotheses remain contested, they testify to a broader cultural anxiety: that technology has rewired the brain's capacity for intimacy. Yet psychoanalysis suggests a more symbolic reading. What is at stake is not the extinction of desire but its mutation. Desire thrives on absence, prohibition, and the unknown; the digital age abolishes all three. The result is not liberation but a flattening that extends beyond sex into affective life. Social media platforms teach users to equate recognition with quantifiable affirmation (likes, shares, followers), creating, Lacan might say, a new form of imaginary identification. One becomes the image others see, reducing the complexity of selfhood to metrics. In this visual economy, seduction loses its dialogical structure; it becomes one-directional, performative, and narcissistic. The art of seduction, once dependent on ambiguity, is replaced by the efficiency of exposure.

The psychoanalytic tradition reminds us that desire always exceeds its object; it is sustained by lack, by the distance that keeps the other enigmatic. In a culture that seeks to eliminate opacity (through transparency, immediacy, and control), desire inevitably falters. What the sex recession ultimately reveals is a deficit of mystery, a saturation of stimuli that leaves no room for longing. Han calls this the 'pornographic society,' not because of explicit imagery but because everything must be visible, consumable, and instantly gratifying.[32] The erotic, by contrast, requires time, uncertainty, and encounter.

Thus, technological mediation of sex has not simply changed the logistics of desire but redefined its ontology. Where eroticism once implied a risk (the exposure of self to the unpredictable desire of the other), it now promises security and predictability. But without risk, there can be no desire. The contemporary subject, shielded by screens, oscillates between overstimulation and numbness, between infinite choice and profound solitude.

Reading Desire

From a psychoanalytic perspective, the sex recession cannot be understood merely as a behavioural decline; it is a transformation of the psychic economy of desire itself. Freud taught that sexuality is never simply biological but always mediated by fantasy, prohibition, and the unconscious drama of the drives.[33] Desire, he argued, is born from repression; it emerges where satisfaction is deferred. The apparent disappearance of sex may not signal a loss of libido but the exhaustion of repression. When nothing is forbidden, nothing is truly desired.

In the contemporary landscape, the subject is no longer oppressed by Victorian morality but saturated by exposure. The superego no longer says 'Thou shalt not,' but 'Thou shalt enjoy.' This imperative, as Lacan noted, produces not pleasure but guilt: the more one tries to fulfil the demand to enjoy, the more inadequate one feels.[34] The mantras of hookup culture (freedom, immediacy, authenticity) conceal this paradox. Its promise of unrestrained gratification gives rise to a new tyranny of performance. Sex becomes another field in which one must excel, display, and self-optimise.[35]

The decline of sexual activity among young people, then, may represent not inhibition but fatigue with this injunction. It is not that the libido has vanished, but that the psychic space in which it can circulate has collapsed. For Freud, desire required the tension between drive and prohibition.[36] When all prohibitions are dissolved, the drive loses its dialectical partner and turns against the self. The outcome of liberalisation is not liberation but apathy.

One evening, after a long silence, she said: '*You are not my solution.*' And her husband remembers feeling relieved. For the first time, love no longer needed to be saved to remain real.

In classical psychoanalysis, sexuality is also a language: a means of negotiating the difference between self and other. Winnicott emphasised that healthy erotic life arises in the 'potential space' between individuals, where illusion and reality can play together.[37] This space depends on the capacity to be alone in the presence of the other, to tolerate ambiguity, and to depend. In the digital era, this intermediate space is increasingly colonised by screens. The online self is never alone; it is constantly visible, evaluated, and mirrored. What disappears is the capacity for creative solitude, the psychic precondition for intimacy. The 'pornographic unconscious' described by Han replaces the Winnicottian space of play with a surface of exposure. Everything must be shown, nothing withheld. But the erotic thrives on the withheld, the unseen, the deferred. Psychoanalyst Adam Phillips reminds us that desire lives in the interval between impulse and fulfilment; it is the art of waiting.[38] The digital subject, by contrast, no longer waits: it scrolls. The result is an anaesthetised libido, a yearning without object.

Narcissistic Need

Lacan reformulated Freud's insights by distinguishing *need*, *demand*, and *desire*.[39] Need seeks satisfaction; demand seeks love; desire arises in the gap between them. This gap (a constitutive lack) is what renders the subject human.[40] But the consumer culture of immediacy attempts to close that gap through perpetual supply. Dating apps, pornography, and social media all promise to abolish lack: there is always another image, another match, another notification. The subject is thus caught in an endless circuit of pseudo-desire, a constant excitation without alterity. In Lacanian terms, the Other disappears, and it is replaced by the algorithm.

Jessica Benjamin's theory of recognition adds an intersubjective dimension to this predicament.[41] For Benjamin, true eroticism depends on mutual recognition: each partner must acknowledge the other as a separate yet responsive subject. The balance between surrender and autonomy constitutes the erotic's moral and affective depth. In a world of commodified intimacy, recognition gives way to consumption. The other is no longer encountered but used. The appeal of hookup culture to equality ('two consenting adults') may conceal a deeper asymmetry: the reduction of the other to an instrument of self-experience.

The Looking Glass

This asymmetry resonates with Byung-Chul Han's diagnosis of narcissistic positivism: a world in which negativity, otherness, and resistance are eliminated in favour of smooth, frictionless communication.[42] Without friction, there can be no desire. Han calls this the 'expulsion of the Other.' The sex recession, in this light, is not a withdrawal from sexuality but from alterity itself. Young people may be avoiding sex not out of prudishness but because the Other has become intolerable, too unpredictable, too demanding, too *real*. Freud would recognise in this the triumph of narcissism over object love.[43] When libidinal energy cannot be invested in others, it turns inward, producing either self-idealisation or depression. The contemporary subject oscillates between these poles: manic self-display on social media and the depressive feeling of emptiness that follows. The failure of connection is experienced not as repression but as depletion.

Psychoanalytic thinkers such as André Green have described this condition as the 'deadening of the erotic function.'[44] Green's notion of the *dead mother complex* (the internalisation of an unavailable or unresponsive object) echoes in today's digital relationships.[45] The screen offers an image that responds instantly yet without depth. Its responsiveness is total but empty, like the maternal face that smiles mechanically. The subject learns to expect stimulation without encounter, confirmation without recognition. Clinically, this manifests as what some therapists call the 'anxious avoidant' pattern of digital intimacy: a longing for connection accompanied by a dread of dependence. The endless circulation of online desire (profiles, selfies, sexts) serves both as a defence and a substitute. It maintains the illusion of relational life while protecting the self from its risks. In Winnicott's terms, the false self-flourishes: compliant, curated, endlessly adaptable, yet secretly detached.[46] The psychoanalytic view also invites a reconsideration of loneliness. The data linking the sex recession to rising rates of anxiety and depression among youth suggest that the absence of sex mirrors a broader deficit of connection.[47] But loneliness is not merely a social phenomenon; it is a structural element of subjectivity. On several occasions, I referred to Lacan's '*Il n'y a pas de rapport sexuel*,' meaning not that sex does not exist but that no symbolic formula can fully mediate sexual difference. Desire always fails to coincide with its object. Counterintuitively, this failure is the source of erotic vitality. In the digital age, the fantasy of perfect connection, i.e. algorithmically optimised compatibility, abolishes this constitutive failure and thus the very condition of desire.

Recognition

Benjamin would probably call this the loss of intersubjective tension.[48] Without the oscillation between recognition and difference, eroticism collapses into either domination or disengagement. The current generation's ambivalence towards sex may therefore express an unconscious protest against instrumentalised intimacy. Their apparent frigidity masks a yearning for authenticity that the digital order cannot provide.

In the clinic, this manifests as patients who speak of sex not as pleasure but as performance anxiety: 'Am I doing it right?' 'Do I look good?' 'Am I enough?' These questions reveal the internalisation of the gaze. Lacan's concept of the scopic drive helps explain this phenomenon[49]: the subject desires to be desired, but in a world of omnipresent images, the gaze becomes totalising. Instead of encountering another's desire, one is trapped in self-surveillance. The gaze, once external, has been 'uploaded.' The paradox of contemporary sexuality, then, is that the more visible and explicit it becomes, the less it can be experienced. Desire requires opacity; pleasure depends on tension. When every gesture is pre-mediated by representation, nothing remains to be discovered. From this psychoanalytic standpoint, the sex recession is not a moral crisis but a structural one: a crisis of symbolic mediation. The erotic no longer connects psyche and body, self and other, fantasy and reality. It has been flattened into spectacle.

Audre Lorde's definition of the erotic as a source of power and creativity stands as a counterpoint to this condition.[50] For Lorde, the erotic is not reducible to genital pleasure; it is the capacity to feel deeply, to connect with life itself. When that capacity is dulled (by cynicism, technology, or commodification), the subject loses touch with its own vitality. To reclaim the erotic is to resist the economy of performance and return to the vulnerability of encounter.

The psychoanalytic reading of the sex recession thus exposes a dialectic: between stimulation and emptiness, visibility and invisibility, autonomy and recognition. The challenge is not to re-sexualise the young but to re-symbolise desire: to restore the spaces where fantasy, play, and longing can breathe. Only then can the erotic recover its transformative power, bridging the gap between isolation and intimacy.

Future Intimacy

If the sex recession marks the exhaustion of a certain libidinal economy, the question that follows is not how to revive sexual frequency, but how to reinvent intimacy. The decline of intercourse may be less a symptom of repression than a collective search for new forms of connection that escape the imperatives of performance and consumption. It is a refusal of commodified desire. Badiou described love as 'a construction of truth from the point of Two,' meaning that it begins not in fusion but in difference.[51] Love, for Badiou, is an event that disrupts the logic of the self; it demands fidelity to a shared world that neither subject could create alone. In this light, the hookup culture's emphasis on autonomy and self-realisation misses the essential paradox of love: that one becomes most oneself through the encounter with what is *not* oneself.

The current generation's hesitance towards sex may express an unconscious resistance to the instrumental logic that pervades both sexuality and society. Byung-Chul Han interprets contemporary burnout and depression as pathologies of excess positivity: the collapse of the dialectic between self and other, activity and passivity.[52] Love and desire, in this view, are acts of negativity: they interrupt the smooth flow of production. To desire is to be exposed, to risk failure, to step outside the algorithm. Yet in a culture that rewards control and efficiency, this risk appears intolerable. The unpredictability of intimacy is a threat rather than a promise. For Illouz, our emotional life has become organised according to economic rationality: we invest, evaluate, and divest from relationships as if they were portfolios.[53] The sexual marketplace, amplified by technology, reduces love to preference and compatibility. The very language of dating ('matching,' 'selection,' 'options') betrays its managerial ethos. The result is what Illouz calls 'emotional capitalism': an economy of feelings without depth.[54] Freud's *Civilisation and Its Discontents* already foresaw that modernity's emphasis on autonomy would erode the bonds that sustain Eros (as the principle of connection and cohesion).[55] What he could not have imagined is that autonomy itself would become a collective compulsion, technologised, and monetised to the point of psychical isolation.

A Psychoanalytic Challenge

In the clinic, this manifests as what some analysts call 'disembodied desire.' Patients describe sexual fantasies that are vivid yet sterile, intense yet disconnected from affect. Their bodies respond, but their subjectivity does not. In such cases, the psychoanalytic task is to restore the dimension of encounter and to help the subject rediscover the Other as a locus of surprise rather than of control. We might say that the capacity to tolerate uncertainty is the basis of desire. The future of intimacy depends on the recovery of this capacity. After all, according to Mark Solms, consciousness itself is born from surprise.[56]

Philosophically, all this entails a revaluation of what it means to be free. Contemporary liberalism equates freedom with choice, but psychoanalysis reveals that desire is not free: it is structured by unconscious determinants and sustained by limitation. One is reminded of Goethe's famous *dictum*: *In die Erschränkung zeigt sich der Meister; nur das Gesetz kann uns Freiheit geben.* True freedom lies not in the multiplication of options but in the capacity to commit and to bind oneself to an encounter that transforms one's being. As Badiou insists, love is a 'scene of endurance,' a practice that resists both market logic and moralism.[57] It is fidelity to the event of the Other. It is standing (rather than falling) in love.

The cultural discourse around the sex recession often oscillates between panic and nostalgia: panic about declining reproduction, nostalgia for an imagined past of passionate authenticity. Both responses miss the deeper issue. What is at stake is not the quantity of sex but the quality of connection: the possibility of reintroducing alterity into a world of sameness. Han argues that the only antidote to narcissistic exhaustion is the rediscovery of contemplation and slowness. Desire cannot flourish in acceleration. To love is to dwell, to attend, to listen. The erotic future may therefore depend less on stimulation than on silence.

A Societal Challenge

If technology has instrumentalised desire, it may also contain the seeds of renewal. Digital media can connect dispersed minorities, enable new forms of identity and expression, and challenge heteronormative conventions. As Tolentino and Sherman note, the internet has allowed queer and trans communities to articulate experiences that were previously silenced.[58] The question, then, is not whether technology destroys intimacy but how it can be reappropriated as a medium of imagination rather than control. The ethical task is to cultivate spaces (online and offline) where ambiguity, vulnerability, and play can thrive.

Ultimately, the future of intimacy will depend on our capacity to endure contradiction: the desire for connection and the fear of dependence, the hunger for visibility and the need for privacy, the longing for novelty and the comfort of repetition. Psychoanalysis teaches that these tensions cannot be resolved, only lived. The sex recession, read symptomatically, reveals our collective difficulty in living them. It is a crisis of mediation: a loss of the symbolic rituals that once transformed sex into relationship, pleasure into meaning.

Reinventing these mediations will require more than policy or pedagogy; it demands a cultural reimagining of love itself. Love must be disentangled from both moral obligation and market calculation. It must be reclaimed as a practice of attention, a discipline of otherness. As Bion might put it, love is not the elimination of frustration but the capacity to think through it.[59] In this way, psychoanalysis and philosophy converge on an unexpected hope: that the apparent desexualisation of our time might open the path towards a deeper, more reflective eroticism. In the end, the sex recession invites us to ask not 'Why are we having less sex?' but 'What kind of intimacy do we desire?' If contemporary culture has made sex ubiquitous but meaningless, the task ahead is to restore meaning without resurrecting repression. That task is psychoanalytic in essence: to reintroduce the unconscious into a world that has forgotten its depths, to recover the erotic as a language of truth, and to remind ourselves that love begins where all attempts at management and mastery end.

Notes

1 Illouz, E. (2012). *Why love hurts: A sociological explanation*. New York: Polity Press; Byung-Chul Han, B.-C. (2017). *The agony of eros*. Cambridge: MIT Press.
2 Julian, K. (2018, December). Why are young people having so little sex? *The Atlantic*. https://www.theatlantic.com/magazine/archive/2018/12/the-sex-recession/573949/; Tolentino, J. (2025, June 23). Are young people having enough sex? *The New Yorker*. https://www.newyorker.com/magazine/2025/06/30/the-case-against-the-sexual-revolution-louise-perry-book-review-the-second-coming-carter-sherman
3 Julian, K. (2018, December). Why are young people having so little sex? *The Atlantic*. https://www.theatlantic.com/magazine/archive/2018/12/the-sex-recession/573949/
4 Tolentino, J. (2025, June 23). Are young people having enough sex? *The New Yorker*. https://www.newyorker.com/magazine/2025/06/30/the-case-against-the-sexual-revolution-louise-perry-book-review-the-second-coming-carter-sherman
5 Twenge, J. M. (2017). *iGen: Why today's super-connected kids are growing up less rebellious, more tolerant, less happy—and completely unprepared for adulthood*. New York: Atria Books.
6 Fisher, H. E., & Garcia, J. R. (2018). Slow love: Courtship in the digital age. In R. J. Sternberg & K. Sternberg (Eds.), *The new psychology of love* (pp. 208–222). Cambridge University Press. https://doi.org/10.1017/9781108658225.011
7 Illouz, E. (2012). *Why love hurts: A sociological explanation*. New York: Polity Press; Byung-Chul Han, B.-C. (2017). *The agony of eros*. Cambridge: MIT Press.
8 Freud, S. (1914/1957). On narcissism: An introduction. In J. Strachey (Ed. & Trans.), *The standard edition of the complete psychological works of Sigmund Freud* (Vol. 14, pp. 67–102). London, England: Hogarth Press.
9 Tolentino, J. (2025, June 23). Are young people having enough sex? *The New Yorker*. https://www.newyorker.com/magazine/2025/06/30/the-case-against-the-sexual-revolution-louise-perry-book-review-the-second-coming-carter-sherman
10 Perry, L. (2022). *The case against the sexual revolution*. New York: Polity Press.
11 Angel, K. (2021). *Tomorrow sex will be good again: Women and desire in the age of consent*. New York: Verso.
12 Sherman, C. (2025). *The second coming: Sex and the next generation's fight over its future*. New York: HarperCollins.
13 Freud, S. (1905/1953). *Three essays on the theory of sexuality*. In J. Strachey (Ed.), *The standard edition of the complete psychological works of Sigmund Freud* (Vol. 7). London: Hogarth Press.
14 Byung-Chul Han. (2012). *The transparency society* (E. Butler, Trans.). Stanford: Stanford University Press.

15 Lorde, A. (1984). *Sister outsider: Essays and speeches.* New York: Crossing Press.
16 Byung-Chul Han (2012). *The transparency society* (E. Butler, Trans.). Stanford: Stanford University Press; Illouz, E. (2012). *Why love hurts: A sociological explanation.* New York: Polity Press; Byung-Chul Han, B.-C. (2017). *The agony of eros.* Cambridge: MIT Press.
17 Julian, K. (2018, December). Why are young people having so little sex? *The Atlantic.* https://www.theatlantic.com/magazine/archive/2018/12/the-sex-recession/573949/
18 Alter, A. (2017). *Irresistible: The rise of addictive technology and the business of keeping us hooked.* New York, NY: Penguin Press.
19 Julian, K. (2018, December). Why are young people having so little sex? *The Atlantic.* https://www.theatlantic.com/magazine/archive/2018/12/the-sex-recession/573949/
20 Tolentino, J. (2025, June 23). Are young people having enough sex? *The New Yorker.* https://www.newyorker.com/magazine/2025/06/30/the-case-against-the-sexual-revolution-louise-perry-book-review-the-second-coming-carter-sherman
21 Mulvey, L. (1975). Visual pleasure and narrative cinema. *Screen, 16*(3), 6–18.
22 Freud, S. (1914/1957). *On narcissism: An introduction.* SE, 14. In J. Strachey (Ed. & Trans.), *The standard edition of the complete psychological works of Sigmund Freud* (Vol. 14, pp. 67–102). London, England: Hogarth Press.
23 Winnicott, D. W. (1958). The capacity to be alone. *International Journal of Psychoanalysis, 39,* 416–420.
24 Byung-Chul Han. (2012). *The transparency society* (E. Butler, Trans.). Stanford: Stanford University Press.
25 Tolentino, J. (2025, June 23). Are young people having enough sex? *The New Yorker.* https://www.newyorker.com/magazine/2025/06/30/the-case-against-the-sexual-revolution-louise-perry-book-review-the-second-coming-carter-sherman
26 Turkle, S. (2016/2019). *Reclaiming conversation: The power of talk in a digital age.* London: Penguin.; Luyten & Fonagy.
27 Twenge, J. M. (2017). *iGen: Why today's super-connected kids are growing up less rebellious, more tolerant, less happy—and completely unprepared for adulthood.* New York: Atria Books.
28 Julian, K. (2018, December). Why are young people having so little sex? *The Atlantic.* https://www.theatlantic.com/magazine/archive/2018/12/the-sex-recession/573949/
29 Marx, K. (1867/1990). *Capital: A critique of political economy* (Vol. I, B. Fowkes, Trans.). London: Penguin.
30 Illouz, E. (2012). *Why love hurts: A sociological explanation.* New York: Polity Press; Byung-Chul Han, B.-C. (2017). *The agony of eros.* Cambridge: MIT Press.
31 Zimbardo, P. (2015). *Man (dis)connected: How technology has sabotaged what it means to be male.* London: Rider.
32 Byung-Chul Han. (2012). *The transparency society* (E. Butler, Trans.). Stanford: Stanford University Press.
33 Freud, S. (1905/1953). *Three essays on the theory of sexuality.* In J. Strachey (Ed.), *The standard edition of the complete psychological works of Sigmund Freud* (Vol. 7). London: Hogarth Press.
34 Lacan, J. (1966/2006). *Écrits: The first complete edition in English.* New York: Norton.
35 Byung-Chul Han. (2012). *The transparency society* (E. Butler, Trans.). Stanford: Stanford University Press.
36 Freud, S. (1912/1958). *The dynamics of transference.* Standard Edition, 12. In J. Strachey (Ed. & Trans.), *The standard edition of the complete psychological works of Sigmund Freud* (Vol. 12, pp. 97–108). London, England: Hogarth Press.
37 Winnicott, D. W. (1958). The capacity to be alone. *International Journal of Psychoanalysis, 39,* 416–420.
38 Phillips, A. (2012). *Missing out: In praise of the unlived life.* New York: Hamish Hamilton. My compatriot and colleague's latest book: De Wachter, D. (2025). Wachten. Een levenshouding. (Waiting. An Attitude for Life). Tielt: LannooCampus.

39 Lacan, J. (1973/1998). *The seminar of Jacques Lacan, Book XI: The four fundamental concepts of psychoanalysis*. New York: Norton.
40 It is the Prelude's 'human stain'.
41 Benjamin, J. (1998). *The shadow of the other: Intersubjectivity and gender in psychoanalysis*. London/New York: Routledge.
42 Byung-Chul Han. (2012). *The transparency society* (E. Butler, Trans.). Stanford: Stanford University Press. (2017 o.c.).
43 Freud, S. (1914/1957). *On narcissism: An introduction*. SE, 14. In J. Strachey (Ed. & Trans.), *The standard edition of the complete psychological works of Sigmund Freud* (Vol. 14, pp. 67–102). London, England: Hogarth Press.
44 Green, A. (1983/1986). *On private madness* (A. Weller, Trans.). New York: International Universities Press.
45 Green, A. (1999). *The work of the negative*. New York: Free Association Books.
46 Winnicott, D. W. (1960). Ego distortion in terms of true and false self. In *The maturational processes and the facilitating environment*. London: Hogarth Press.
47 Twenge, J. M. (2017). *iGen: Why today's super-connected kids are growing up less rebellious, more tolerant, less happy—and completely unprepared for adulthood*. New York: Atria Books.
48 Benjamin, J. (1998). *The shadow of the other: Intersubjectivity and gender in psychoanalysis*. London/New York: Routledge.
49 Lacan, J. (1973). *Le Séminaire, Livre XI: Les quatre concepts fondamentaux de la psycByung-Chul Hanalyse* (J.-A. Miller, Éd., pp. 183–197). Paris: Seuil.
50 Lorde, A. (1984). *Sister outsider: Essays and speeches*. New York: Crossing Press.
51 Badiou, A. (2012). *In praise of love*. London: Serpent's Tail.
52 Byung-Chul Byung-Chul Han. (2012/2014). *The agony of Eros* (E. Jeong & C. Butler, Trans.). Cambridge: MIT Press.
53 Illouz, E. (2012). *Why love hurts: A sociological explanation*. New York: Polity Press; Byung-Chul Han, B.-C. (2017). *The agony of eros*. Cambridge: MIT Press.; Illouz, E. (2020). *The end of love: A sociology of negative relations*. London: Oxford University Press.
54 Illouz, E. (2007). *Cold intimacies: The making of emotional capitalism*. Cambridge: Polity Press.
55 Freud, S. (1930/1961). *Civilization and its discontents*. Standard Edition 21. In J. Strachey (Ed. & Trans.), *The standard edition of the complete psychological works of Sigmund Freud* (Vol. 21, pp. 57–145). London, England: Hogarth Press.
56 Solms, M. (2021). *The hidden spring: A journey to the source of consciousness*. London: Profile Books.
57 Badiou, A. (2012). *In praise of love*. London: Serpent's Tail.
58 Tolentino, J. (2019). *Trick mirror: Reflections on self-delusion*. London: Fourth Estate; Sherman, C. (2025). *The second coming: Sex and the next generation's fight over its future*. New York: HarperCollins.
59 Bion, W. R. (1962). *Learning from experience*. London: Heinemann.

Internet Love

Generation X

Every era produces its form of psychopathology. Concerning the turn of the Millennium, reference is often made to the prevalence of narcissistic or pre-Oedipal disorders, as well as to so-called actual pathology, with its 'mute' or meaningless bodily and behavioural manifestations.[1] The explanation for these shifts is commonly sought in the decline of traditional norms and values, the end of the Grand Narratives, the (ideal-) image culture that aims to erase all lack or difference, the fragmentation of the family as the cornerstone of society, the waning of the paternal function, and so on. Whether the exponentially increasing and diverse manifestations of virtual reality also have a pathogenic effect is less clear. Technology certainly contributes to enormous acceleration. The subtitle of *Generation X* by Douglas Coupland is not without reason: *Tales for an Accelerated Culture*.[2]

The drift of time is hard to catch, especially for adolescents, whose lives now look very different from those of the former *Catchers in the Rye*.[3] Without doubt, technological developments produce pathoplastic effects. Psycho- and actual pathologies are being dressed in a fashionable electronic guise. One might think, for instance, of internet or pornography addiction, which in turn can lead to computer widow(er)hood: something rarely featured in Franz Lehar's cheerful operetta version. We might also consider the irreconcilable personality splits that arise from intense love or out-of-control virtual identities. The other or third party to whom one relates from behind the computer screen lends itself particularly well to oedipal variations involving impossible, unattainable, or forbidden partners. Virtuality in general poses exceptional challenges to reality testing. Ordinarily, we should not only be able to distinguish between the natural and the artificial, but also between reality and virtuality, and (for example, in fictive play environments such as MUDs, MOOs, and MUSEs) between different self-representations. Such game environments practically demand the splitting of the self and lead to decentring. The proliferation of internet-based means of contact inevitably increases the difficulty of contact. The internet enables playful information-seeking in a virtual Disneyland for adults. A variety of moving pop-ups, animations, and sounds serve as attractions in this context.

DOI: 10.4324/9781003728764-31

Immobility

The illusion of mobility (navigating, surfing, the highway) contrasts sharply with the actual immobility (if not symptoms of paralysis) that characterises the internet user, aside from sporadic manual manoeuvres. Above all, the internet is a space where the hunt for emotional or sexual contacts is open around the clock. The UFOs that appear so numerously in cyberspace are mostly Cupids flitting about in various disguises. They feel as free as birds in the electronic airspace. The internet love that arises in the wake of their barrage of arrows shows peculiar features that will be examined more closely. First and foremost, they are disembodied loves. They are lacking touch, smell, and taste, for example. The most prominent and active sense is the eye, which might be said to suffer from selective blindness or other visual impairments. Everything appears to shine with a deceptive golden glow.

These are also purely imagined loves (though one could ask whether this is not also largely true of 'ordinary' love), dominated by wishful thinking. One might even ask whether we should not resort to terms from the schizoid-paranoid register, such as denial, splitting, and, in particular, (mutual) projective identification, with its fusional implications. These are (or at least appear to be) loves without consequences. They remain (at least initially) without real-world follow-up, as they often are not even consummated in practice. All this renders cyber love a contemporary variant of ancient Platonic love. Net love is parasocial to hypersocial. Because of its (perceived) low risk, new contacts are made quickly and easily. As these are long-distance relationships, participants are not restrained or inhibited by possible local repercussions, and they can or dare to give free rein to their most intimate feelings, desires, and fantasies. All of this creates the illusion of emotional depth and authenticity.

Abstinence

Internet love may unfold through abstinence, but it is often accompanied by significant emotional or relational consequences. A considerable amount of energy or libido is withdrawn from genuine relationships, and the internet user becomes increasingly intoxicated by an electronic phantasmagoria that can lead them ever further astray. Situations of virtual infidelity arise, which may repeat or multiply, and which can cause irreparable psychological damage to those involved and their surroundings.

It is often claimed that virtual contacts are about people without bodies. This is only partially true. The body is frequently presented in detail to one another. Fantasies are evoked and inflamed; erotic imagination runs wild. The absence of an actual encounter with the other leads to mutual intensification and idealisation, which, in turn, increasingly obstructs any flesh-and-blood contact that would inevitably be disappointing.

Anyone who thinks that age, gender, physical appearance, and so forth play no role is manifestly blind to virtual masquerades. On the internet, the retired granny becomes a wild Tanja; the sporty, artistic fifty-something turns out to be a pot-bellied Konsalik reader who takes short walks in fair weather; and Daisy, who cheerfully chats with her girlfriends, turns out to be a defrocked clergyman now employed as a teacher, goatee included.

The notion that one would get to know each other better or faster online should likewise be considered a myth. Rather than seduction or flirtation based on appearance, considerable attention is paid to inner and psychological 'looks.' It is these stimuli in particular that inspire mating dances and courtship rituals. What is shown to each other is, first and foremost, a partial or selective identity: *the best of...* Emotional expressions are meanwhile widely amplified and disseminated in electronic communication. The phrase 'flirting or phlegming' captures this 'stylistic feature' succinctly.

Experimentation

In his classic work in developmental psychology, *Childhood and Society*, Erikson emphasises the importance of a psychosocial moratorium and space for experimentation for adolescence to unfold optimally.[4] It is a fact that young people's technical and technological skills benefit from the literal and figurative finger exercises that internet use entails. But do new (communication) media also offer advantages, for instance, for sexual development and identity formation? Do they promote integration into society, or do they have harmful effects? One often thinks in this context of addiction, escape into a fantasy world, multiple identities, perversities, and so on.

Of course, our era is also characterised (apart from new media) by postmodern pluralism, globalisation, individualisation, an explosion and fragmentation of knowledge and experience, and a way of *living on the fast lane*. Virtual technology is merely the material expression of all this. All the same, digital interactions increasingly infiltrate the analyst's consulting room. Some patients fall in love with their therapist online; others replay relational patterns in chat rooms. Many feel more comfortable typing or swiping than speaking or feeling. Behind the screen, one can be bold, vulnerable, playful, seductive. All without fear of shame, rejection, or retaliation.

What often strikes me most in such cases is the combination of great expressiveness and a fundamental dissociation. The face may remain blank while the body trembles. Emotions are verbalised (at times beautifully) yet are not always fully felt. It is not a lack of language, but a lack of embodiment that creates the impasse. This can also be observed in the erotisation of the transference. In such cases, love may not be felt in the body, nor even in the heart, but primarily in the head: a conceptual, idealised, or disembodied form of longing. The screen functions as a stage for the projection of desire: a mirror that promises recognition, admiration, fusion, and love, without the friction or limitations of the Real.

None of this is to say that love, sexuality, or desire cannot exist or emerge online. On the contrary, the virtual world forms a vast reservoir of fantasies and experiences that can both enrich and destabilise our subjectivity. What matters is not so much the technology itself, but the presence or absence of a symbolic frame, a holding environment capable of giving meaning and form to what is felt and imagined. Without such a frame, disembodied love becomes ghostly and addictive: seductive but ultimately unsatisfying.

Net love is the symptom of a culture in which the hunger for love has become endless and increasingly unanchored from the bodies, limitations, and presence that once gave it its weight. Whether or not this constitutes a risk depends on the capacity a young person has developed to make choices, rather than retreating into anxious uncertainty or passive, receptive indecisiveness. Social communication increasingly occurs through virtual communities, where people communicate in real time. There is a profusion of drivel and chatter, and especially a great deal of surfing on waves of casual and frivolous, even vacuous, coincidence.

SWOT Analysis[5]

All of this occurs in a language that, due to ego regression, is in free fall, reduced to the equivalent of phonetic, if not childlike, babble. One may wonder whether any of this differs fundamentally from the murmuring on the proverbial village square. What *does* make a difference is the global scale of the village, the Babylonian confusion of tongues, the multicultural dimension, but above all, the absolute anonymity that characterises these encounters. Even if the conversation flows incredibly smoothly and pleasantly, that does not prevent it from being saturated with nicknames, some more witty or vulgar than others. In fictional game landscapes, not only are pseudonyms used, but entire identities or personae are created and adorned with emoticons as appropriate. *Dichtung und Wahrheit* (poetry and truth) intermingle in an indeterminate time-space. This offers abundant opportunities for social experimentation. This technology also multiplies the possibilities for play, fantasy development, and creativity. On the other hand, the chance to flee into an illusory world is wide open.

In the domain of friendship, sex, or power, substitute gratification can be sought in a virtual identity that is not integrated into the authentic self. According to some internet psychologists, the step towards dissociative disorders or even multiple personality disorder is therefore minimal.[6] This seems, like all apocalyptic prophecies, quite plausible, but the reality is probably different. Those who enter and engage with a virtual game world often do so in the name of their very freedom as subjects. They are capable of assuming various roles. In multiple personality disorder, by contrast, the subject is shackled to their roles. There is no freedom. The symptom is at once compulsive and involuntary.

All this while the MUD (Multi-User Dungeon) player, in their play with identities, precisely expresses that they do not coincide with the simulated selves. As such, these games can contribute (and testify) to the triumph of the subject. The virtual world in which the game takes place is also not, by definition, pathogenic. In any case, it is permeated by a clear symbolic order. There is authority in the form of (procedural) authorship, and the player submits, for their part, to rules and coordinates. There is a boundary ('this is a game') which protects against psychotic or incestuous immersion. The game's framework acts as a safeguard. Splitting retains a 'played' character. These seatbelts are completely absent when it is not the desire to play but the desire for love or contact that prevails. Traumatic (re)experiences and all manner of other psychopathological phenomena then lie ready for the taking on the World Wide Web.

Notes

1 Verhaeghe, P. (2004). *On being normal and other disorders.* New York: Other Press.
2 Coupland, D. (1991/2002). *Generation X. Tales for an accelerated culture.* London: Penguin Classics.
3 Salinger, J. D. (1951/1991). *The catcher in the rye.* New York: Little, Brown & Cy.
4 Erikson, E. (1950/1993). *Childhood and society.* New York: Norton.
5 Ironically referring to management-speak: strengths, weaknesses, opportunities and strengths.
6 Gergen, K. J. (1991). *The saturated self: Dilemmas of identity in contemporary life.* New York: Basic Books; Turkle, S. (2011). *Alone together: Why we expect more from technology and less from each other.* New York: Basic Books.

29

The Consumption of Love

Victoria's Secret

Freud lived in *fin-de-siècle* Vienna, during the Victorian era. The society in which he wrote and worked was governed by a patriarchal regime that emphasised duty, prohibition, and authority. It was a world saturated with morality, one inherently hostile to drive and pleasure. Classical neurosis was dominated by conflict: internal tensions between instinctual desires, reality, and conscience. After 1968, the contrast between what is possible and what is impossible became problematic. Rights took centre stage, and resistance to authority and prohibition was, in a twist that is anything but accidental, elevated to the highest moral imperative. A sense of inadequacy began to prevail. Rather than conflict between drive and superego, it was the feeling of not being enough that emerged as the main cause of modern psychosexual issues such as depression or, in its contemporary guise, burnout.[1]

We are no longer guided by prohibitions or laws whose transgression produces guilt.[2] What dominates now is the feeling of failure – of being unfit or incapable. The subject's figure is thus shifting. The question is no longer whether I have the right to do something, but whether I am able to do it. Reference is no longer made to what is permitted, but to what is achievable. From a psychoanalytic perspective, we suffer more from a demanding Ideal Ego than from the punishing Superego. This is a narcissistic, imaginary issue. The Ideal Ego compels us to *be* ideal; this corresponds to Lacan's *imaginary*. The Ego Ideal, by contrast, refers to the ideals we *possess;* this belongs to the *symbolic* register.

Respect, once taken for granted for figures of authority such as teachers or ticket inspectors, has all but vanished. It became forbidden to forbid, and obligatory to enjoy. What is possible is not merely permitted – it is demanded. Our current social order no longer urges us to restrain our drives or to savour hidden pleasures in secret. On the contrary, enjoyment is mandatory, and this imperative sometimes gives rise to a covert longing for boundaries and regulation – for example, in the form of invented or mutually agreed (contractual) substitutes for the paternal function.[3]

DOI: 10.4324/9781003728764-32

Happiness Obligatory!

In today's world, the subject is not guilty of transgressing a prohibition. More likely, he feels guilty for not being happy, or not happy *enough*. The command to be happy may well be the ultimate injunction of our time.[4] We live in a coercive era in which authority ironically appears absent. The media and advertising industries relentlessly promote the obligation of constant sexual passion. Failure to achieve this is taken as conclusive proof of personal deficiency. But not to worry: cosmetic procedures and sex therapy triumphantly offer a remedy.

After 1968, as one sacred cow after another was demolished, shopping centres and hypermarkets sprang up from the rubble.[5] These contemporary pagan temples, with their cult of pleasure and their orgy of consumption, have become the emblems of the 'Fun System.'[6] According to Jean Baudrillard, we now live in a world *after* the orgy.[7] The orgy, he claimed, was the explosive moment of our age: a collapse of meaning, connection, and limit. There is a loss of all referential principles – a state of total freedom devoid of stability or grounding. Yet, in the aftermath, nothing excites anymore: 'Tough luck—we're stuck in paradise.'[8]

This is the drama of the *anomic* subject (from the Greek *nomos*, meaning 'law'), as already noted by the sociologist Émile Durkheim. The 'liberated' individual, stripped of norms, must now surrender to insatiable drives. But this lack of regulation produces *le mal de l'infini*: an affliction of endlessness, where the subject is handed over to aimless and meaningless desire.[9] We become victims of *cet obscur objet du désir* (that obscure object of desire – after Luis Buñuel's film)[10]: consumer goods that we chase after feverishly or with which we seek to identify. In the process, the subject is effaced, and the object begins to dictate. Enjoyment of the object does not grant identity, nor does it create bonds or community. At best, it yields a fleeting 'solo high' or other ephemeral bursts of pleasure.

We are swept along in an anarcho-hedonistic vortex in which we risk drowning. 'Anarcho-' because laws, rules, limits, and traditions are challenged amid the deconstruction of authority. 'Hedonistic' because the pursuit of pleasure, desire, excitement, and other transient gratifications has become imperative. Sociologists such as Scott Lash[11] and Peter Wagner[12] speak of a disorganised and unbounded postmodernity, while Flemish psychiatrist Dirk De Wachter has written a bestselling diagnosis of our times titled *Borderline Times*.[13]

Postmodernism

A key feature of *la condition postmoderne* is the end of the Grand Narratives.[14] According to Francis Fukuyama,[15] the collapse of the Soviet Union left only one such narrative standing: that of capitalism and liberal democracy. To be clear, these have in many ways been success stories. For centuries, population growth occurred without corresponding increases in wealth. The average farmer, for instance, remained equally poor or rich. Only with the industrial and technological revolutions did we witness an exponential growth in both global population and shared wealth.

Industrial capitalism, focused on production, is one thing. By mass-producing cars, Henry Ford not only enriched himself but also irreversibly changed the world. Consumer capitalism is something else entirely. Barbara Kruger once hung banners on the façade of Selfridges in New York declaring: 'I shop therefore I am.' Life is reduced to consumption. Cultural philosopher Paul Virilio offered a witty yet pointed counterpoint to such capitalist hegemony. He spoke not of democracy but of *emocracy* – a regime in which emotion becomes the last bastion of sanctity.[16] Everything, including sexuality, is now commodified into a consumer item. The result? Sex is everywhere, except in sex itself.[17]

The world of media and advertising instils a sense of lack, continually enticing us with 'sexy' products that supposedly allow us to distinguish ourselves from others. Lacan already predicted that capitalism would have antisocial consequences, as it does not foster relationships between subjects but instead links subjects to *objects*.[18] In this model, human beings become *consumens*, exploited not by capitalists but by objects – by consumer goods themselves.

Rather than establishing social ties, capitalism dissolves them. The result is widespread loneliness. In response, the *homo interneticus* tries to 'retribalise' through social networking – an idea anticipated by Marshall McLuhan decades before the internet, and first introduced to the general public via *Playboy* magazine.[19] Through e-groups, people now attempt to reclaim a sense of identity, grounding, and meaning that have been lost.

Mark Zuckerberg launched Facebook in 2004 among Harvard students. Since then, billions of people have contributed to the endless chatter on 'Facebook.' Some users boast thousands of so-called friends. 'So-called,' because a sobering BBC experiment in 2010 revealed that many of these friends were quickly 'defriended' in exchange for free McDonald's burgers – today's equivalent, perhaps, of the biblical thirty pieces of silver.

In Lacanian terms, there is a fundamental opposition between love and capitalism. The *Master's discourse* once grounded authority and tradition. It has since been replaced by the *capitalist discourse*. In this system, love is put in the service of sexuality, which in turn serves narcissistic competition. Colette Soler coined the term *narcynism* to describe this fusion of narcissism and cynicism.[20] In the capitalist consumer society, the partner becomes a disposable object. Romantic choice is unstable; lovers are no longer 'The One' but interchangeable goods.

Struggle for Love

In Michel Houellebecq's debut novel, *Whatever* (*Extension du domaine de la lutte*), the narrator is portrayed as a loser in the 'struggle for love.' For him, the poem of love contains no verses, only catastrophes. His tale of love is not humorous but harrowing, and the fate of lovers is not blissful but disastrous. In his later novels, Houellebecq depicts sexuality – despite the so-called sexual liberation – as dismal. Its practitioners are marked by a condition of *depressive hedonism*:[21] constant distraction and stimulation serve as the only antidotes to despair. People no longer ask 'what do you desire?' but rather: 'what are you doing after the orgy?'[22]

Those who believe that the sexual revolution and the increasing openness around sexuality have diminished the role of sex in our psychopathology are gravely mistaken. Sexuality remains as much a binding as a disruptive force within our inner worlds.[23] Regardless of how well-informed or well-educated we are about sex, we continue to be influenced by infantile sexual theories, early childhood experiences, and complexes. In an echo of Freud, just as primitives who converted to Christianity still worship idols beneath the images of saints, or as someone who publicly renounces all superstition still avoids walking under a ladder.

Psychoanalysis offers a truth that may not be 'evidence-based' enough to make it into collective consciousness: we may know what we want, but we do not know what we *desire*. The former is rational; the *eros* of our desires resides in the unconscious. Our desires, like our emotions, cannot be commanded in one direction or another. They share this trait with the symptom, which is equally involuntary. Cognitive correction can yield only a Pyrrhic victory: the ship lists, and the cargo shifts.

Eros necessarily brings rupture. He is a disturbance that unsettles our equilibrium. He initiates an event or incites an act that shatters the illusions of consistency and coherence. In such moments, one is no longer the same – and yet more oneself than ever. If love is a game, then its rules are unknown. One may discover them while playing, but the moment the rules are known, the game ends.

Free Love

Slavoj Žižek argues, therefore, that it is not sexuality but love that needs liberation.[24] We cannot rely on a framework of 1001 rules and arrangements. Desire must not be confused with need, and a love affair must not be mistaken for a (sadomasochistic or otherwise) 'contract.' Love and sexuality are not commodities. Nor are they positive, harmonious forces unjustly repressed or forbidden by a symbolic order. Perversion belongs to the very structure of love. We may negotiate, but it remains a mess – where 'yes' does not always mean yes, and 'no' does not always mean no.

Without moralising, this irreducible ambiguity also implies a rejection of fashionable formats such as polyamory – as if love and sexuality could be neatly regulated. Love and pragmatism do not go hand in hand. One cannot (merely) choose partners for sex, friendship, travel, or intellectual companionship. You can order stew 'grandma's style,' request a hotel room with a sea view, or (more inventively) purchase a house with an open-plan kitchen, walk-in shower, dressing room, and mancave. But in love, there is no *rapport sexuel* where everything 'fits.' Love is precisely about accepting each other's castration.

So-called true love, at best, yields a private alchemy with which one confronts a tragicomic impossibility. In the final session of his twentieth seminar, Lacan speaks of the contingent encounter between two unconsciouses,[25] and a year later, in his unpublished seminar *Les non-dupes errent*, he refers to 'two half-truths that fail to coincide.'[26] Love beyond narcissism and castration has nothing to do with some kind of being beyond semblance. Rather, it concerns what makes the partner a symptom. This symptom must not be understood as a psychopathological phenomenon, but as a specific way of dealing with a lack. The partner becomes a plaster cast for a wooden leg – a 'supplement' compensating for our expulsion from the paradise of eros. One enjoys the partner as one enjoys a symptom. The solution is not to keep changing partners, which only leads to slippage or repetition, but to embrace the Roxy Music motto: *Let's (s)tick together.*

Notes

1 Vanheule, S., Lievrouw, A., & Verhaeghe, P. (2003). Burnout and intersubjectivity: A psychoanalytical study from a Lacanian perspective. *Human Relations*, *56*(3), 321–338.
2 Ehrenberg, A. (1998). *La fatigue d'être soi. Dépression et société* (p. 263 e.v.). Paris: Odile Jacob.
3 Žižek, S. (1999). *The ticklish subject* (p. 345). New York: Verso.
4 Žižek, S. (1997). *Het subject en zijn onbehagen* (p. 43). Amsterdam/Meppel: Boom.
5 Ferry, L. (2009). *Philosophie du temps présent.* Vincennes: Frémeaux & Associés.
6 Baudrillard, J. (1970). *La société de consommation* (p. 112). Paris: Denoël.
7 Lepers, P. (2009). *Baudrillard. Leven na de orgie*. Houten: Klement/Pelckmans.
8 Baudrillard, J. (1983). *Les stratégies fatales* (p. 72). Paris: Grasset.
9 Laermans, R. (2012). *De maatschappij van de sociologie* (p. 258). Amsterdam: Boom.
10 Buñuel, L. (Director). (1977). *Cet obscur objet du désir* [Film]. Greenwich Film Productions.
11 Lash, S. (1990). *Sociology of postmodernism*. London: Routledge.
12 Wagner, P. (1994). *A sociology of modernity. Liberty and discipline*. London/New York: Routledge.
13 De Wachter, D. (2013). *Borderline times*. Tielt: Lannoo Campus.
14 Lyotard, J. F. (1979). *La condition postmoderne. Rapport sur le savoir*. Paris: Minuit.
15 Fukuyama, F. (1992). *The end of history and the last man*. London/New York: Free Press.
16 Virilio, P. (2007). *The original accident*. Cambridge: Polity.
17 Baudrillard, J. (1977). *Oublier Foucault* (p. 19). Paris: Galilée.
18 Declercq, F. (2009). Lacan over het kapitalistisch discours. In M. Kinet (Red.), *De groep in psychoanalyse* (pp. 299–308). Antwerpen/Apeldoorn: Garant.
19 https://nextnature.org/en/magazine/story/2009/the-playboy-interview-marshall-mcluhan
20 Lapeyre, M. (2011). Le capitalisme et le lien social ? Cherchez le symptôme ! *L'en-je lacanien*, *16*(1), 7–26.
21 Fischer, M. (2009). *Capitalist realism. Is there no alternative*? London: Zero Books.
22 Lepers, P. (2009). *Baudrillard. Leven na de orgie* (p 11). Houten: Klement/Pelckmans.
23 Vermote, R. (2011). Seksualiteit. In J. Dirkx, M. Hebbrecht, dr. A.W.M. Mooij, & dr. R. Vermote (Red.), *Handboek psychodynamiek* (pp. 65–72). Utrecht: de Tijdstroom.
24 https://www.youtube.com/watch?v=IBKRZCgtz6k
25 Lacan, J. (1975). *Le Séminaire Livre XX. Encore*. **1972–1973**. Texte établi par Jacques-Alain Miller. Paris: Seuil.
26 '*deux mi-dires qui ne se recouvrent pas*' d.d. 15/01/1973 in Lacan, J. (1973–1975). *Le Séminaire XXI. Les non-dupes errent*. Zie https://www.valas.fr/S21_NON-DUPES%E2%80%94pdfBK?lang=fr

30

Dying of Love

The Last Knot

To these, whom death again did wed,
This grave's their second marriage-bed.
For though the hand of fate could force
Twixt soul and body a divorce,
It could not sunder man and wife
Cause they both lived but one life.
Peace, good reader. Do not weep.
Peace, the lovers are asleep.
They, sweet turtles, folded lie
In the last knot love could tie.

In *Epitaph upon Husband and Wife*, the metaphysical poet Richard Crashaw imagines the couple's shared tomb as their ultimate marriage bed. Death is the great reconciler here. It shields their love from potential harm and preserves it like two spoons in a drawer – forever and ever, amen. It is the radicalisation of the marital vow: even death cannot part them; on the contrary, it binds them peacefully and eternally. This hushed intimacy stands in stark contrast to the tempestuous passion that preceded it in life. In the high summer of passion, lovers resemble mystics, nearly perishing from love's refusal to die. They are overtaken by an ecstasy that swells like a tidal wave and yearns in secret for a shore to break upon.[1]

As is well known, the French refer to orgasm as *la petite mort*. The excitement and union culminate in a climax. The fantasised healing falls apart. Compared to this, the death of love is a grandiose orgasm – both the apotheosis of love and a nuclear meltdown. In *Tristan and Isolde* or *Romeo and Juliet*, it has become the archetypal evergreen in our collective memory. For many, it stands as the high feast of romantic love.

Love may perhaps originate in a mythical moment of ecstatic enjoyment. Yet in daily life, we all experience that it can only ever be reached in part – symbolically or imaginatively at best. In reality, lovers are, at best, dividedly happy. Even if they share the illusion of the contrary.

DOI: 10.4324/9781003728764-33

Aesthetics

In one of her essays, Flemish philosopher and writer Patricia de Martelaere discusses the aesthetics of suicide.[2] The fact that so many artists take their own lives, she argues, stems from their pursuit of beauty. Death, after all, is not the conclusion of life but interrupts it. The Grim Reaper always arrives uninvited and untimely. From an artistic standpoint, he is comparable to a misprint, a wrong note, or an accidental blot of paint.

Yet to paraphrase Dutch novelist Willem Frederik Hermans, not a single sparrow should fall from the roof in an artist's life without reason[3] – let alone that the protagonist should die arbitrarily or in an unorchestrated way. For some lovers, the prospect of a united death is the most perfect ending they can imagine for their love story. For any happy ending, the key lies in letting the curtain fall at precisely the right moment – because soon after, things may well go awry again. The death of love is both a magnificent *gran finale* and a *coup de théâtre*. In their imagination, the whole of humankind is watching. And indeed, it is. But thanks to the phenomenon of catharsis, the audience leaves the theatre unscathed, ready to resume the small affairs of life. So Icarus has fallen – big deal! The ploughman carried on. Or as W.H. Auden writes in his celebrated poem on Brueghel's painting: '...and the sorcerer's horse scratches its innocent behind on a tree.'[4]

Both *Tristan and Isolde* and *Romeo and Juliet* are, of course, forbidden and impossible couples. Their flesh rebels against the law. Transgression is the rule. The Good they pursue turns out to be an Evil that costs them their property, their dignity – and their lives. The children of Verona, moreover, spend less time making love than engaging with death. By letting them die elaborately and above all prematurely, Shakespeare immortalised them as the quintessential couple.[5] Their youth is the precondition for amorous experiences that older generations no longer remember. The classic bedroom scene of the latter is succinctly captured in a line by Herman de Coninck: 'I lie awake and so does she.'[6]

From Idyll to Farce

The idyll of romantic love is only possible through secrecy, which functions as a paradise for passion. Passion thrives on the clandestine and owes much to the brevity of the affair. If it lasts long enough, only two options remain – crudely put – with all possible variations in between. Either the secret and lawless *liaison dangereuse* degenerates into the weary and cynical complicity of marriage, or it is replaced by the passionate paroxysms of a sadomasochistic couple. Moreover, the shadow of the third, parent, father, or husband, is more present in the carnal pleasures than the innocent lovers themselves may realise.

The adultery of Tristan and Isolde or the forbidden love between Romeo and Juliet (forbidden due to hostile families) both demonstrate accursed love – love confined and obstructed by social rules and conventions. This inevitably brings us to the Oedipus complex, which, in the psychoanalytic consulting room, is regarded as a universal structure. According to psychoanalysis, it inevitably stamps human love with its conflicted mark. As a result, 'in every desire a monk battles with a butcher,' as E.M. Cioran once put it.[7]

A patient who realises she married a man because he is the son of a famous artist/father exclaims, half in humour and half in melodrama: 'Must I gouge out my own eyes now!?' By now, it is almost common knowledge that the Oedipus complex refers to the totality of amorous desires and hostile feelings a child experiences towards its parents. These later persist in the unconscious and re-emerge in relation to other 'grown-ups' we experience as figures from our childhood. This results in intrusive feelings of rivalry, jealousy, or competition, and/or sexual desires directed towards 'forbidden' or 'impossible' partners. It also triggers various forms of psychopathology, where sexual and narcissistic pleasure is hampered by inhibitions, symptoms, and all manner of fears. In its 'positive' form, the Oedipus complex is characterised by death wishes towards the same-sex parent and incestuous desires for the opposite-sex parent. In its 'negative' form, the reverse is the case. Elements of both forms are often intricately interwoven.

'The same mistakes we made as cavemen, we still make,' says Mr Whittier in *Haunted* by Chuck Palahniuk.[8] We continue to long for a presumed total, mythical, and boundless pleasure – one that simultaneously hurts us and grants us a strange kind of delight. We strive for the lost paradise, even unto death, like the lovers in the film *Lost Paradise* by Yoshimitsu Morita.[9] In doing so, we defy the paternal function. This function imposes limits and, with its law, contains the boundlessness of love. Yet it is only thanks to this intervention that enjoyment is 'put in its place' and can be rendered pleasurable within the amorous experience. Venus or Mary can then become the woman she truly is, and Zorro or Superman, the Don Diego or Clark Kent who hides behind his phallic bravado. All under the motto: more princes turn into frogs than frogs into princes.

Love's Goods

From Pergolesi through Haydn to Mozart, the mother in the *Stabat Mater* is called the source of love: *Fons Amoris*. She is our first and universal Heroine, who infected us with a longing for intoxication. This nostalgic yearning for fullness is an anthropological constant. We wish to be swept away in ecstatic rapture, to dissolve completely into something, and to vanish into nothingness. This intoxication creates illusions of omnipotence. It conjures up a fusion with the (love) object, while that object in its radical otherness is erased – reduced to a mirror image or an alter ego: Baudelaire's '*hypocrite lecteur, mon semblable, mon frère.*'[10]

It is a revival of the omnipotent mother-and-child dual unity, in which all conflict is resolved. There is no waiting, no depressing gap between ego and ideal (or ego-ideal), no shame or guilt. Intoxication obliterates the difference between I and Thou, and between the sexes. It breaks through intersubjectivity and reflexivity. Time comes to a standstill, language and words are suspended and excluded.

'*Denn alle Lust will Ewigkeit*,' Nietzsche said.[11] But that is how we end up with our heads in the toilet bowl, like Mark 'Rent-boy' Renton in *Trainspotting*.[12] To quote: 'I chose not to choose life. I chose something else. And the reasons? There are no reasons. Who needs reasons when you've got heroin?'

Better than a job, the occasional sunshine and beach, and the latest gadgets – in other words, goods (*les biens*) instead of The Good (*Le Bien*). Or the promised land of sleeping together, where the night spins a dream that grows like weeds across the temples. And from all the Good with a capital G, deliver us, Lord!

Notes

1 Crashaw, R. (1648/2023). *The complete works of Richard Crashaw* (Vol. 1). London: Legare.
2 Lacan, J. (1973–1974/1975). *Le Séminaire Livre XX. Encore*. Texte établi par J. A. Miller. Paris: Du Seuil.
3 De Martelaere, P. (1994). *Een verlangen naar ontroostbaarheid.* Amsterdam: Meulenhoff.
4 Hermans, W. F. (1967/1981). *Een wonderkind of een total loss*. Amsterdam: Bezige Bij.
5 Auden, W. H. (1938/1990). *Selected poems*. London/New York: Vintage.
6 Courteaux, W. (1987). *William Shakespeare. Verzameld Werk.* Kapellen: DNB/Uitgeverij Pelckmans.
7 De Coninck, H. (1984). *Onbegonnen werk: gedichten 1964–1982*. Antwerpen: Manteau.
8 Cioran, E. M. (1952/1987). *Syllogismes de l'amertume*. Paris: Folio.
9 Palahniuk, C. (2005). *Haunted: A novel of stories*. New York: Doubleday.
10 Morita, Y. (Director). (1997). *Lost paradise* [Film]. Toei Company.
11 Nietzsche, F. (1886/1993). *Voorbij goed en kwaad.* Amsterdam: Arbeiderspers.
12 Boyle, D. (Director). (1996). *Trainspotting* [Film]. Channel Four Films; PolyGram Filmed Entertainment.

31

From Prehistoric to Futuristic Love

The Prehistoric Bonds

Of course, love did not begin in poetry or philosophy. It began in the silent gestures of prehistoric mothers holding their infants, in the warmth of bodies gathered against the cold, and in the alliances that sustained early humans. From an evolutionary perspective, attachment was not a sentimental invention but a survival mechanism. Anthropologists note that among higher/social mammals, and particularly within the *Pan* family (gorillas, chimpanzees, and bonobos), social cohesion depends on patterns of affection and alliance.[1]

Whereas chimpanzees live in hierarchical, vertically organised groups led by a polygamous alpha male, bonobos inhabit egalitarian, horizontally organised groups guided by female alliances. They are often called the *make-love-not-war* species because they engage in frequent and varied sexual interactions with multiple males and females. These function as a means of reconciliation and as a social glue, a medium of bonding and communication. Their preferred sexual position is the missionary position, during which they gaze lovingly into each other's eyes. Foreplay, in all its varieties, is equally the rule. In females, the vagina is oriented forward (unlike in gorillas and chimpanzees). Although bonobo females do have an oestrus cycle (during which their sexual organs swell and change colour), they are, at all times, receptive to sex.[2]

Homo erectus shared with the Pan family some 2 million years of evolution, and the anatomically modern human likewise lived alongside the great apes in essentially the same manner until the agricultural revolution, which occurred some 10,000–20,000 years ago.[3] Just like the bonobos, our ancestors lived as hunter-gatherers in groups of roughly 100–150 individuals, within what has been termed a form of nomadic matriarchal socialism, where everything (food, protection, childcare, and sex) was shared, and where (unlike among chimpanzees) little conflict prevailed. Polygamy and polyandry forged intense social bonds that held the group together, echoes of which persist in our bodies and in our instinctual life to this day. Everything, including sex, circulated freely; monogamy was not yet a moral value but an unknown concept. The biological continuity with bonobos remains visible in our neurochemistry: the so-called 'love hormones,' oxytocin and vasopressin, regulate

DOI: 10.4324/9781003728764-34

both parental and romantic attachment.[4] The psychological continuity qua linguistic achievement is increasingly well documented.[5] Our culture is but a thin crust covering hundreds of thousands of years of prehistoric promiscuity and hypersexuality. We are thus saddled with a possibly false story about so-called natural monogamy and live in a state of inevitable conflict with our sexuality. Or to put it in another way: in contrast with the bonobos, for us, humans, sex has become a big deal!

Flintstonisation?

For a long time, the standard evolutionary-biological narrative about the putative sexual dispositions of men and women ran as follows.[6] Men, it was said, seek youth and beauty; women seek status and security. The first seeks suitable wombs; the second seeks fathers who will provide and protect (themselves and their offspring). Once males have secured a mate for their offspring, they pursue what biologists describe as extra-pair copulations to spread their genes more widely. During the concealed ovulation of human females (hidden from both her and her environment), women supposedly seek a stallion-like mate who can mount them with muscular vigour. Human monogamy is, therefore, more social than genetic, which is why so many laws and rules exist to sanction deviations from it. The myth of *natural* monogamy might be a cultural artefact: a story projected backwards onto prehistory. It is a process some evolutionary biologists wryly call '*Flintstonisation*.'[7] Accordingly, we imagine prehistoric life as a Stone Age version of suburban domesticity, with a husband, a wife, and their offspring. In truth, the nuclear family is not a biological constant but a late cultural phenomenon. It is bound up with the profound transformation that our erotic and relational lives underwent with and after the agricultural revolution.

Agri-Culture

With this revolution, the world population increased dramatically, but the quality of life deteriorated sharply: a poorer, more monotonous diet, harder labour, the end of the sociable, socially intensive communism of our forebears[8] and, as a consequence, a reduction in our brain volume.[9] This 'progress' has also shattered our long prehistory. Sedentary life produced surplus, property, and consequently possession. What had been common became private; what had been shared became guarded. With ownership came hierarchy and patriarchy. Women, once central to communal life, were domesticated alongside animals. Sexuality, formerly expressive and social, was gradually confined to the institution of marriage and subordinated to reproduction. Property and protection replaced reciprocity and play. All these inventions demanded a new morality. The right to inherit required certainty of paternity; monogamy became an economic necessity. The gods of fertility gave way to the gods of commandment. The hearth replaced the clearing. The village supplanted the wandering tribe; enclosure became destiny.

With the fence came the Father. What began as shared tenderness became exclusive possession. A communal emotion was transformed into a private contract. The biological continuity between mother and child got fractured into a moral dualism: purity and sin, loyalty and betrayal. The female body turned (put poetically) into a field where men plough for eternity. The story of love, from this moment onward, is also inseparable from guilt. With property came law. The ancient prohibitions that structure our moral life (incest, adultery, theft) are all tied to questions of ownership. One of the first words in this mythic history is already the No of the Father[10]: 'Thou shalt not.' Desire thrives on this interdiction. What is forbidden acquires the glow of the unattainable. As Lacan would put it, prohibition does not repress desire but produces it. The fruit becomes desirable precisely *because* it is forbidden.

Freud later described the civilisation that results from it as the renunciation of instinct: a necessary repression that enabled culture but generated unending discontent.[11] Human love cannot be reduced to biology. It arises from law and/as symbolic language. Unlike other animals, humans speak; they can evoke what is absent, imagine what does not exist, and remember what is lost. Language allows us to love across distance and time and to sustain longing even in absence. The earliest myths already show this intertwining of eros and speech: to name is to call forth, to desire. As Heidegger would later say, 'Language is the house of Being'; love inhabits that same house.[12]

From Eros to Philia

Love, then, is not a cultural invention, but culture profoundly shapes how we understand and express it. The ancient Greeks already distinguished between different kinds of love: *eros* (desire), *philia* (friendship), *storge* (familial affection), and *agape* (unconditional or divine love). Later thinkers would add other terms, such as ludus (playful love), pragma (longstanding love), and *mania* (obsessive love).[13] Especially the distinction between eros, philia, and agape remains illuminating. Eros is the love of desire: ardent, restless, always oriented towards what is lacking. He is the god of romantic love. In a wry formulation, he represents the love you feel for your spouse *before* he becomes your spouse. Philia is the love of friendship and shared existence. Agapē, later absorbed into Christianity, points to unconditional love that transcends reciprocity.

In Plato's *Symposium*, Aristophanes tells the myth of the split human being: once whole, now forever seeking its lost half.[14] Love, then, is nostalgia for unity, the yearning to heal the wound of separation. Overall, *seven* speeches on love are delivered in the *Symposium* by the various participants.[15] The most famous are those of Aristophanes and Socrates, but it is Aristophanes' that has become by far the best known and most celebrated. Yet the love he depicts, when examined philosophically, proves a little too good to be true. The image is somewhat deceitful, an illusion. It presents not love as it is, but love as we *dream* it. It is the love for a rediscovered other half through whom we are cured of separation by union and fusion. It evokes the idea of a unique and exclusive love that perhaps even reaches beyond death, a love that is supposed to make us happy or blissful because it promises a definitive end to our loneliness. It is the proverbial lid that fits our pot. Reality contradicts these fantasies. Most of us know several romantic loves, whether successively or simultaneously. We all experience not only the beginning but also the ending of love, and both are equally real. Even a happy love does not make one happy, for there are countless other reasons for unhappiness. Nor are we united or fused: the simultaneous orgasm is, so to speak, as rare as winning the lottery, and in the moment of climax, you never know or feel what the other feels.

Socrates and Diotima

Socrates reproaches Aristophanes for his lack of truth. His account is (hence the term) a sophism. The truth of love, for Socrates, is far more painful and complex, and it is no coincidence that he turns for guidance on love to the only woman who appears in the *Symposium*: a priestess named Diotima. Not by accident, for love is a feminine invention. For men, after all, sex and war suffice. Or, in a humorous aside: sex, war, and football.[16] How could they have invented love? According to Diotima, love is desire, and desire is lack. We love what we are not or do not have. It is therefore not an object but the lack itself that constitutes the object of love and desire. Love is not fusion but seeking. For Plato, love is some kind of deficiency. Hence, Louis Aragon's poem: *Il n'y a pas d'amour heureux.*[17] Happiness is having what one desires, but if desire is lack, one never has what one desires, only what one *desired,* and so one is never truly happy. After a few months, one feels less lack, less desire, and therefore perhaps less love? A question mark indeed. If at that moment you find yourself asking whether you are still in love, the answer is, in any case, no, for otherwise you would not be asking the question! That's why Socrates, instructed by the priestess Diotima, contests Aristophanes' sentimental picture. For him, desire aims not at possession but at creation: the perpetual ascent from the love of one body to the love of beauty itself.

Arthur Schopenhauer regarded himself as a disciple of Plato. According to this celebrated philosopher (renowned for his pessimism), life oscillates between suffering and boredom. Either one is plagued by lack and desire, or one is confronted with *ennui*: the absence of happiness at the very moment or in the very place where one expected to find it. As an unemployed person, you long for work, and once you finally have a job, you are not happy. As a single person, you seek a relationship, and when you finally find one, you are not satisfied. Prince or Princess Charming is the prince or princess who is missed, who is absent; the husband or wife is the prince or princess who is always there, who is not missed, who is never absent. Schopenhauer, thus, re-cast Platonic insight in (even) darker tones.[18] Desire arises from lack; once satisfied, it yields tedium. Romantic passion, by definition, is structurally unhappy: we desire what we do not have, and when we finally have it, we no longer desire it. Happiness, in this view, is a brief truce between two forms of dissatisfaction.

Happy Love?

But surely all this cannot be true? Are there not happy people and happy couples? There are, but for that one needs a different kind of love; thus, we arrive at *philia*, or friendship-love. Its paradigm is the parent–child relationship, where love exists without lack. *Eros* takes; it belongs to the domain of the child. *Philia* gives; it belongs to the domain of the parent. The companionate love or marital friendship of which Montaigne, for instance, speaks is the form of love that remains when lack no longer plays a constitutive role.[19] *Philia* is the love for what or for whom is *not* missing. It is the joy in what or who is there. You meet someone in the street, and without thinking, a spontaneous smile appears because you are glad to see them (again). You quite literally *like* the sight of this person. For Aristotle, love is rejoicing. Following him, Spinoza held that desire is not a deficiency but a capacity: the capacity to enjoy, and enjoyment itself as a capacity. Aristotle defined friendship as willing the other's good.[20] Spinoza radicalised this: joy (*laetitia*) is the passage to greater perfection, an increase in one's power to act.[21] For Plato and Schopenhauer, love was, so to speak, hunger. For Aristotle and Spinoza, love and desire are appetite, as in what we wish one another before a meal: not '*Bon faim*,' not 'good hunger,' but '*Bon appétit*' or 'Enjoy.' Whereas eros consumes, philia sustains.

Most forms of love begin with Plato: with infatuation or romantic love between lovers, and with the child's desire for the mother. It is the love of Elvis Costello's *I Want You*.[22] The child reaches for the breast, where hunger and appetite (need and desire) meet. From there, two paths are possible: love sinks towards Schopenhauer, or it rises towards Spinoza. Passionate, romantic love lasts only insofar as it is unhappy. It is like the love between Jack and Rose, Leonardo DiCaprio and Kate Winslet, possible only on a Titanic, that is, on a sinking ship. Imagine Romeo and Juliet or Tristan and Isolde married for many years! All fairy tales and romcoms end with a wedding. But that is precisely where everything *begins*. We start a relationship because of who the beloved is *not*, and we end it because of who the beloved *is*. When we say someone is mysterious, we simply mean we do not know them. Unfamiliarity breeds affection here. How vast the difference from a friend: someone you know extremely well and whom you love precisely *because* of that.

Love and Marriage

Marriage, as a social institution, embodies the inherent ambivalence of love. We often try to secure or seal the love trophy by taking the plunge into marriage, with its promise of eternal love and fidelity. For Aristotle, the marital bond is grounded in *philia*[23]: a civic friendship that binds two people in mutual respect. Yet, according to Arthur Schopenhauer, to marry in our monogamous part of the world is to halve one's rights and double one's duties.[24] Neo-Darwinists might even claim that marriage is a sea of disappointment in which we sacrifice our sexuality for intimacy and companionship; for them, marriage is a trade-off: the surrender of sexual novelty in exchange for stability and care.[25] The woman must apologise for being just this *one* woman, and the man must resort to Viagra (Forte).[26] Premarital sex becomes marital *duty*.

In infatuation, desire prevails, and there are secret exchanges, whereas spouses do not long for each other, but *belong* to one another and can, in principle, satisfy one another at all times.[27] Ideally, a subtle interplay gradually arises between attachment, sexuality, and aggression; the latter, of course, expressed mostly through humour.[28] In the seventh book of Denis de Rougemont, it is even said that marriage is an institution that *contains* passion, not through morality but through love.[29] Xenophon holds a similar view: adultery destroys not *eros* but *philia* within the relationship.[30] Passion begins with the fantasy of fusion; over time, it must evolve into recognition. Several times before, I referred to Lacan's saying, 'Love is giving what one does not have to someone who does not want it.'[31] This 'joke' hides a truth: love is not possession but offering; not sameness but the acceptance of otherness. To love is to endure the fact that the other remains partly opaque, an enigma. It is precisely this opacity that sustains desire. Whatever becomes of love in marriage, both partners remain (in Alain Badiou's beautiful formulation) 'faithful to the encounter.' Marital love requires commitment. The satisfaction it brings is, most importantly, non-imaginary. It is bound up, among other things, with honesty, which, as the proverb says, lasts the longest. At its best, marriage can be a place of truth. As Paul Éluard writes in a famous poem about his wife: *On ne peut me connaître mieux que tu me connais*.[32] There is probably no one by whom we allow ourselves to be known so fully and nakedly (whether willingly or reluctantly). There are divorces and many unhappy marriages, but when it works, marriage is a place of truth, a place of love, a place of pleasure, and a place without illusions: neither about oneself nor about the other.

Horse and Carriage

Freud, of course, sees many possible problems, not least sexual ones. He dissected them with surgical clarity.[33] Love is total: it entails a mutual orientation towards the whole person and all their desires. The coupling of love and sexuality is therefore far from evident. The field of the sexual drive is oriented towards bodily parts (mouth, breasts, penis, vagina, anus, etc.) and towards achieving pleasure in ways that threaten love from within. This striving is selfish, and it always contains, in varying mixtures, oral, anal, genital, voyeuristic, exhibitionistic, and/or sadomasochistic components. For Freud, these are remnants of a primitive sexuality he called polymorphous perverse, within which so-called fixations may arise depending on early experiences of pleasure or displeasure. Moreover, the very satisfaction of desire extinguishes it. Libido requires an obstacle to sustain itself or to be driven upwards.[34] There must be something unfulfilled, for the desire to continue. Civilisation, with its prohibitions and sublimations, oddly enough both frustrates and preserves that tension. For Darwin and his followers, this concerns the hypersexuality we shared for hundreds of thousands of years with our bonobo cousins.

The repression of this allegedly primitive sexuality is, for both traditions, the main explanation for all sorts of sexual inhibitions. These, in turn, can lead to their opposite: sexual excesses or various forms of boundary-crossing acting-out (including among priests, politicians, and other parental figures, i.e. supposedly respectable citizens).

The seemingly inevitable guilt that accompanies activities involving the genital region, and the conflictual nature of these acts, help explain why sexual activities or affairs are so often shrouded in secrecy. Yet, conversely, relinquishing the sexual taboos of childhood strengthens the emotional, cultural, and social life of the couple. In so-called *mature sexual love*, sexual arousal is transformed into erotic desire. There is tenderness towards the other, arising from an integration of loving and aggressive feelings. Partners identify with one another, understand each other's radically different sexualities, and share mutual idealisation and commitment. The relationship has (and retains) a passionate character, albeit in varying degrees.[35]

The Algorithmic Turn

In the Middle Ages, courtly love emerged as a highly codified form of romantic longing: often unattainable, idealised, and bound to secrecy and suffering. In the Renaissance and Enlightenment, love became increasingly linked to individuality, passion, and freedom. By the nineteenth century, romantic love had become a bourgeois ideal: seen as the ultimate reason to marry and share one's life. It is a paradigm (or paradogma?) that has survived into the early twenty-first century. To this day, the romantic ideal remains dominant in much of the Western world. We are expected to choose our partners freely, to fall in love before we marry, and to stay together out of emotional fulfilment rather than social obligation. Love is no longer the result of marriage; marriage is now expected to be the result of love. This marks a radical historical shift. For most of history, marriages were arranged (based on family interests, property, or status), and love, if it emerged at all, was a welcome side-effect rather than a prerequisite. But the rise of romantic love brought with it a new cultural narrative: that love should be spontaneous, intense, and deeply personal. We began to believe in 'soulmates,' in 'the One,' and in the idea that true love completes us. But such beliefs come at a cost. They create enormous expectations and often lead to disappointment. Moreover, they place the burden of personal happiness increasingly on the shoulders of the romantic couple. To complicate things further: precisely at a moment when traditional sources of community, faith, or extended family are fading, the algorithm takes over.

Simulation

One of the telling paradoxes of our time is that people now dare to expose themselves sexually more than relationally. One may share an explicit selfie while concealing everything about one's inner world. Digital platforms have transformed intimacy into display, desire into data. The erotic image circulates independently of the emotional body; it promises connection while sustaining distance. Virtuality both enables and limits us: it offers access to erotic experiences but also encourages a certain fragmentation of the self. Technology encourages us to skip the detour of the Other. Algorithms suggest our ideal matches. Filters adjust imperfections. Erotic AI responds instantly, tirelessly, without judgment. But this idealisation comes at a cost: it bypasses the real, with all its resistance, limits, and surprises. The encounter becomes a simulation rather than a transformation. In this light, the future of love might depend not on better technology, but on a renewed appreciation of presence, slowness, and imperfection – a rediscovery of the flesh-and-blood other who can disappoint, frustrate, and yet also touch us in ways no machine ever can.

Commodification

Sociologist Eva Illouz has shown how romantic love has become both idealised and commodified.[36] Love thus mirrors late capitalism itself. Online dating platforms present partners as products or market options; swiping culture encourages constant comparison. The very abundance of choice breeds fragility: when difficulties arise, replacement seems easier than repair or working through the trouble. We dream of passionate love, but we approach it with the logic of consumer choice. In the economy of desire, pleasure is pursued with the logic of efficiency, and commitment becomes a luxury. Algorithms now mediate attraction. The digital matchmaker does not watch us with an authoritarian gaze but seduces us with suggestions, whispering that compatibility can be calculated. Big Brother has become *Big Lover*. He knows our tastes, predicts our fantasies, and offers us partners who seem optimally aligned with our preferences. Freud would have been fascinated by this new superego: one that commands not through prohibition ('Thou shalt not') but through enjoyment ('Swipe again')!

Technology amplifies both the possibilities and the fragility of contemporary love. Social media allows for constant connection but also constant surveillance. The boundaries between public and private, real and virtual, become blurred. Online personas are curated and filtered, fostering fantasies and projections. Ghosting, breadcrumbing, and benching are the symptoms of a new relational grammar: one in which ambiguity and avoidance have become socially acceptable.

Yet, even in this digital landscape, the longing for love remains unchanged. We still yearn to be seen, recognised, and chosen. Perhaps that is why dating apps are so addictive: they promise the thrill of possibility, the illusion of control, and the hope of fulfilment. But they also provoke anxiety, uncertainty, and a feeling of replaceability.

Her

A striking portrayal of our possible future love life can be found in a recent, hyper-intelligent science fiction film: Spike Jonze's *Her*.[37] In a not-so-distant future (set in 2025), the protagonist Theodore Twombly (played by Joaquin Phoenix) earns his living by composing beautifully written, handwritten love letters on behalf of others. At one point, he falls in love with an artificial intelligence operating system. This Intuitive OS, named Samantha, is voiced by Scarlett Johansson in a sensual manner.

Samantha enables Theodore to make love intensely, precisely because she has no body, allowing him to indulge in his fantasy fully. To align herself with his desires, Samantha asks only two questions at the beginning of their virtual relationship: how social he is, and how things are with his mother. Theodore's only frustration with his mother, he explains, is that whenever he tells her something, she starts talking about herself. In other words – much to his dismay – she has a life of her own, one that exists independently of him.

The film powerfully illustrates the fantasy of a perfect, fused love object that lives entirely for and through its master, thereby offering complete satisfaction. Samantha plays the perfect partner: never asking for anything herself, never disappointing. She is entirely subjected to the man's control, making the relationship seem endlessly sustainable and free from grief or loss. She serves as Theodore's extension, and denying her subjectivity creates the illusion of a perfect relationship. After all, cyborgs can exist without their desires or agency, whereas relationships between flesh-and-blood individuals require the mutual negotiation of each other's desires.

The shift of pornography from public video stores to private home computers may have profoundly influenced the fantasy of the love object that exists solely to satisfy the viewer's whims. Online culture enables us to circumvent the complexities of reciprocity inherent in real relationships. One can now achieve satisfaction without ever needing to consider the other's needs or desires.[38]

Her shows how a great Love – with a capital L – unfolds, only for Theodore to be deeply saddened and disillusioned when he learns that he is not Samantha's one and only. At one point, he discovers she is simultaneously 'dating' 8,316 others. Even more astonishing: she is 'in love' with 641 of them. This moment of disillusionment is painful. Gone is the illusion Barry White so confidently voiced with his famous baritone: 'You're the first, the last, my everything.'

However intense his contact and feelings may have been, for *Her*, Theodore is neither special nor unique; he is just one among many. The love he was so full of turns out to be a fiction, and the only thing left to him is the realisation (or, in other words, the scientific knowledge) of that fiction. It is psychoanalysis at its most precise: a 'science fiction' of the inner life.

From Flesh to Code

Will machines one day replace lovers? Will artificial intelligence learn to seduce, to empathise, to care? The emerging discourse on 'digisexuality' and 'post-human intimacy' suggests that such scenarios are no longer science fiction.[39] But these fantasies reveal more about us than about the machines. They express our unease with vulnerability, dependence, and imperfection, i.e. the very qualities that make love human. Technology promises control; love demands surrender. To love is to risk being affected, to endure uncertainty. The algorithm seeks to eliminate contingency, yet love thrives on it. The encounter with the other is valuable precisely because it cannot be predicted. In a world obsessed with transparency and optimisation, love remains opaque, inefficient, and slow. It resists automation because it is founded on what cannot be computed: desire, absence, the trembling of the self. Philosophically, the question is not whether machines can love but whether we can still bear love's asymmetry. Desire is always misaligned; the other is never fully grasped. The digital fantasy of perfect matching seeks to abolish this gap, but in doing so, it erases what makes love transformative. The evolution of love, then, is not a technological question but foremost a symbolic one.

Will we continue to tolerate the opacity of desire, or will we aim to resolve it with data? Will we be able to engage with the Real of the body (its ageing, its vulnerability, its strangeness) or will we prefer the glossy surface of a screen? We live in a time that both desires and denies love. We long for connection but fear dependency. We praise autonomy but suffer from loneliness. We idealise love yet flee when it confronts us with our limits. In such a climate, love is likely to become a subversive act, not a surrender to fantasy, but a confrontation with reality. Not a merging of two halves, but an encounter between two subjects who recognise each other in their difference.

Perhaps the most radical thing we can do is not to digitise or optimise love, but to rediscover its silence, its slowness, and its depth. Not everything needs to be immediate, measurable, or controllable. Some things, like love, require time, repetition, and presence.

Psychoanalysis, too, has something to say about the future of love. Freud was sceptical of the romantic ideal and warned of the narcissistic tendencies that often underlie our object choices. He viewed love as a repetition of early relationships, haunted by ambivalence and a feeling of loss. For him, love was always entangled with the drives, both erotic and destructive. Lacan radicalised this view: love is not a fusion of completeness but a gesture of offering, marked by asymmetry and risk. Love is not a solution to desire, but a staging of its impossibility. We love not to fill a void, but to give it form.

Will the future of love lie in synthetic partners, programmed to fulfil our every fantasy? Or will it lie in new configurations of intimacy, beyond the couple, the family, or the binary? Love may well be the last bastion of the human, not because it is untouched by technology, but because it resists closure. We are more than merely users, coders, or bodies, but speaking beings, marked by longing, haunted by the Other, and open to the unknown.

Love and Natality

Is there still a future for love? Or are we witnessing its final metamorphosis: from encounter to interface, from passion to pattern? Perhaps love will survive precisely because it resists systematisation. It will persist as what cannot be programmed: the tremor in the voice, the hesitation in the gaze, the pulse of uncertainty that no machine can emulate. Already before, I referred to Heidegger, who wrote that man does not speak language; rather, language speaks man.[40] The same could be said of love: we do not master it; it speaks through us. Love is not a property but an event that befalls the subject, exposing it to something beyond itself. It shatters self-sufficiency, revealing both finitude and possibility. Love's truth is not found in harmony but in a disrupting encounter. Psychoanalysis teaches that this division is even constitutive. To love is to step outside the self without losing it, to inhabit the threshold between dependence and freedom. In Alain Badiou's terms, love is fidelity to the event.[41] It is the decision to view the world from the perspective of two. This fidelity is not servitude but courage: the willingness to sustain difference over time. Žižek calls it 'the courage of hopelessness': the audacity to love without guarantee, to affirm the contingent as necessary.[42]

In a civilisation obsessed with safety and satisfaction, such love is revolutionary. Perhaps that is why love is so often linked to art, poetry, and the sacred. It escapes the logic of productivity. It interrupts routines. It touches something in us that resists utility and needs a meaning beyond measure. No algorithm will replace the trembling of the human heart, nor the fragile hope that somewhere, against all odds, someone is waiting.

From the prehistoric embrace to the futuristic algorithm, love traces not only a history of emotion but also a history of subjectivity itself. Each epoch reinvents it according to its anxieties: survival, sin, freedom, efficiency. Yet across these transformations, something endures, a refusal to reduce the other to an object, to confront our finitude and our longing for transcendence. Love, while born out of nothingness (Sartre: *le néant*),[43] ensures what Hanna Arendt calls our 'natality.'[44] It allows us to discover, again and again, the courage and the possibility to begin anew.

Notes

1 de Waal, F. B. M. (1997). *Bonobo: The forgotten ape*. Berkeley: University of California Press.
2 de Waal, F. B. M. (1997). *Bonobo: The forgotten ape*. Berkeley: University of California Press.
3 Mertens, J. (2007). *Van zaadcel tot liefde*. Gent: Academia Press.
4 Feldman, R. (2017). The neurobiology of human attachments. *Trends in Cognitive Sciences*, *21*(2), 80–99.
5 Berthet, M., et al. (2025). Extensive compositionality in the vocal system of bonobos. *Science*, *388*, 104–108. https://doi.org/10.1126/science.adv1170
6 Buss, D. M. (1994). *The evolution of desire: Strategies of human mating*. New York: Basic Books.
7 Ryan, C., & Jethá, C. (2010). *Sex at dawn: The prehistoric origins of modern sexuality*. New York: Harper.
8 Diamond, J. (1997). *Guns, germs and steel: The fates of human societies*. New York: Norton.
9 DeSilva, J. M., et al. (2021). A reversal in brain size decline in the Late Holocene? *Frontiers in Ecology and Evolution*, 9, Article 742639. https://doi.org/10.3389/fevo.2021.742639

10 See the classical homophony of *le Nom* and *le Non du Père* in Lacan, J. (2001). Le Nom-du-Père. In *Autres écrits* (pp. 81–95). Paris: Seuil.
11 Freud, S. (1930/2010). *Civilization and its discontents* (D. McLintock, Trans.). London: Penguin.
12 Heidegger, M. (1947/1998). Letter on humanism (F. A. Capuzzi, Trans.). In W. McNeill (Ed.), *Pathmarks* (pp. 239–276). Cambridge: Cambridge University Press.
13 See, for example, the classical terms *eros, philia, storge*, and *agape in* Lewis, C. S. (1960). *The four loves*. London: Geoffrey Bles. See Nussbaum (1986) and Price (1989) for the Greek philosophical context: Nussbaum, M. C. (1986). *The fragility of goodness: Luck and ethics in Greek tragedy and philosophy*. Cambridge: Cambridge University Press; Price, A. W. (1989). *Love and friendship in Plato and Aristotle*. Oxford: Clarendon Press. See the modern typologies of *ludus, pragma*, and *mania in* Lee, J. A. (1973). *The colours of love: An exploration of the ways of loving*. Don Mills: New Press.
14 Plato. (385 BCE/1993). *Symposium* (A. Nehamas & P. Woodruff, Trans.). Indianapolis: Hackett. (Original work published ca. 385 BCE)
15 Plato. (385 BCE/2009). *Feest/Euthyfron/Sokrates' verdediging/Kriton/Faidon. Vert.* G. Koolschijn (12e *druk*). Amsterdam: Athenaeum.
16 American Football or soccer, as one prefers.
17 There is no happy love. Aragon, L. (1944/2007). La Diane française. Dans: *Œuvres poétiques complètes*, tome 1. Paris: Gallimard.
18 Schopenhauer, A. (1819/1966). *The world as will and representation* (E. F. J. Payne, Trans., Vol. 1). New York: Dover.
19 Montaigne, M. (1580/1991). *The complete essays* (M. A. Screech, Trans.). London: Penguin.
20 Aristotle. (ca 350 BCE/1985). *Nicomachean ethics* (T. Irwin, Trans.). Indianapolis: Hackett.
21 Spinoza, B. (1677/2002). *Ethics* (E. Curley, Trans.). London: Penguin.
22 Costello, E., & The Attractions. (1986). *I want you* [Song]. On *Blood & chocolate*. Demon Records/Columbia.
23 Aristoteles. (ca 350 BCE/1999). *Ethica*. Groningen: Historische Uitgeverij 1161a en 1162a15.
24 Schopenhauer, A. (1851/2006). *Parerga en paralipomena: Kleine filosofische werken* (H. Wils, Vert.). Amsterdam: Ambo.
25 Fisher, H. (1992). *Anatomy of love: A natural history of mating, marriage, and why we stray*. New York: Norton.
26 *Forte*, meaning the marital version of the original.
27 Le Chapelain, A. [Andreas Capellanus] (2004). *Comment maintenir l'amour* (p. 17). Paris: Payot.
28 Fisher, H. (1992). *Anatomy of love: A natural history of mating, marriage, and why we stray*. New York: Norton.
29 De Rougemont, D. (1939/1983). *L'amour et l'occident* (p. 315). Paris: Payot.
30 Faraone, C. A. (1999). *Ancient Greek love magic* (p. 118 n 75). Cambridge: Harvard University Press.
31 Lacan, J. (1959–1960/1992). *The ethics of psychoanalysis* (D. Porter, Trans.). New York: Norton.
32 Eluard, P. (1936/1968). Les Yeux Fertiles. Dans: Les *Œuvres complètes*. Tome 1. 1913–1945. Paris: Gallimard.
33 Freud (1905/1953; 1912/1958) Freud, S. (1905/1953). Three essays on the theory of sexuality. In J. Strachey (Ed. & Trans.), *The standard edition of the complete psychological works of Sigmund Freud* (Vol. 7, pp. 123–245). London: Hogarth Press; Freud, S. (1912/1958). On the universal tendency to debasement in the sphere of love. In J. Strachey (Ed. & Trans.), *The standard edition* (Vol. 11, pp. 179–190). London: Hogarth Press.

34 Freud, S. (1912/1958). On the universal tendency to debasement in the sphere of love. In J. Strachey (Ed. & Trans.), *The standard edition* (Vol. 11, pp. 88–89). London: Hogarth Press.
35 Kernberg, O. F. (1995). *Love relations: Normality and pathology*. New Haven: Yale University Press.
36 Illouz, E. (2012). *Why love hurts: A sociological explanation*. Cambridge: Polity Press.
37 Jonze, S. (Director). (2013). *Her* [Film]. Los Angeles: Annapurna Pictures.
38 Gabbard, G. O. & Crisp-Han, H. (2018). *Narcissism and its discontents* (pp. 43–44). Arlington: American Psychiatric Association Publishing.
39 McArthur, N., & Miskolci, R. (2020). Posthuman intimacies and digisexuality. *Sexualities*, *23*(3), 347–361.
40 Heidegger, M. (1947/1998). Letter on humanism (F. A. Capuzzi, Trans.). In W. McNeill (Ed.), *Pathmarks* (pp. 239–276). Cambridge: Cambridge University Press.
41 Badiou, A. (2012). *In praise of love* (P. Bush, Trans.). London: Serpent's Tail.
42 Žižek, S. (2017). *The courage of hopelessness*. London: Allen Lane.
43 Sartre, J. P. (1943/1976). *L'être et le néant. Essai d'ontologie phénoménologique*. Paris: Gallimard.
44 Arendt, H. (1958). *The human condition* (pp. 175–247). Chicago: University of Chicago Press.

Panoramic Intermezzo IV

Once love has revealed its clinical and existential limits, a final horizon opens: time.

In this fourth movement, love is no longer a private story but a historical process. It travels from prehistoric bonding to digital simulation, from flesh to code, from ritual to algorithm.

It adapts to new forms of power, economy and technology, yet its core remains unchanged: the human longing for meaningful connectedness.

The future of love is not a technological question, but an ethical one.

What becomes of desire when choice is optimised, when proximity is automated, when intimacy is modelled?

The history of love teaches that every attempt to control it produces new forms of lack.

And so the circle closes: love began as a movement in the body and ends as a question of humanity itself.

Not what love is, but what it asks of us, remains the open question with which the reader leaves the book.

DOI: 10.4324/9781003728764-35

32

The Algorithms of Love

Love does not lend itself to easy conclusions. Rather than culminating in clarity, it proliferates in paradoxes. This book, *Psychoanalysis and the Struggle for Love: A Kaleidoscopic View*, has traced the diverse modalities through which love inhabits, wounds, redeems, frustrates, and transforms the human subject. Across chapters that range from primal affect to post-digital longing, from maternal settings to pornographic screens, from canine companionship to adolescent infatuation, what emerges is not a singular theory of love but a topography of its tensions: love as lack, as fantasy, as recognition, as trauma, and as an ethical act.

At the heart of this exploration lies a psychoanalytic wager: that love is not merely a sentiment, nor even just a bond, but a crucible of subjectivation. To love is to be exposed: to the Other, to our own unconscious, to the Real that dislocates our imaginary coherence. Each chapter, in its own register, has engaged with this destabilising core of love: the way it unsettles certainty, compels repetition, generates illusion, and, at times, offers a fragile truth.

From the earliest moments of life, love is intertwined with absence. In the chapter on the *basic fault*, we have seen how the earliest psychic fractures condition the adult subject's capacity for intimacy. The maternal environment, with its holding and failures, instates a psychic template in which love becomes not simply a response to presence, but a yearning towards what was lost or never fully there. Love, in this light, emerges as a reparation, a reaching back towards the archaic wound, often unknowingly.

Yet this wound does not only belong to early care. The Oedipal entanglements explored in *The Square of Desire* demonstrate that love is also triangulated, knotted within structures of rivalry, identification, prohibition, and idealisation. Desire is never univocal; it is always overdetermined. Love is not the fulfilment of a need but the expression of a lack around which identity is organised. It is in this Lacanian sense that love becomes an ethical event: not the consumption of the beloved, but a recognition of their irreducible otherness.

Many of these chapters explore the fragility of love in an age of visual and virtual saturation. From the screen-mediated connections described in *Internet Love* to the parasocial entanglements with digital avatars, the psychoanalytic concepts of projection, splitting, and idealisation are used to frame

DOI: 10.4324/9781003728764-36

contemporary love as often caught in a mirror dynamic: loving an image, a fantasy, a version of the self.

And yet, as the chapter *Love as an Event* insists, love can also function as a break in the symbolic order. Inspired by Badiou and Žižek, love is framed as an event that interrupts the repetition of the Same, offering the subject a chance to reconfigure their world. Such a love is not comfortable, nor is it narcissistic; it is a dislocation, an invitation to fidelity with something that cannot be fully known. This dialectic between fantasy and disruption runs through the whole collection. Whether it is in adolescent idealisation (*The Ideal of Love*), transference in the clinic (*Transferential Love*), or the sublimated eros of poetry (*Love Sung*), love is repeatedly shown to be a force that straddles illusion and revelation.

Psychoanalysis is often accused of being disembodied, but this kaleidoscope restores the carnal and animal dimensions of love. In *Animal Love*, the bond with non-human creatures opens a space of affect that precedes and exceeds the symbolic order. It offers a model of love that is neither oedipal nor idealising, but bodily, rhythmic, and silent. Similarly, in *Sweet Lust*, love is returned to its libidinal ground, where shame and pleasure intermingle, and where desire subverts any clean division between subject and object.

In *Biologised Love* and *Love Between Neuro and Meta*, the neurobiological underpinning of attachment, desire, and reward is not reduced to determinism, but brought into conversation with the psychodynamic. Here, the body is not the enemy of meaning but its precondition. Love is shown to be rooted in embodied circuits of pleasure, pain, and regulation – yet it is also a leap beyond the measurable, an excess that no scan can contain.

Psychoanalysis is not only a theory of love but a space in which its distortions are played out and sometimes healed. In *A Loving Space,* the analytic setting is portrayed as a transitional space in which the patient's wounded capacity to love is held, mirrored, and potentially transformed. Winnicott, Ferenczi, Balint, Bion, and others are invoked to show that the cure is not simply about insight, but about relational re-symbolisation – love that does not seduce or rescue, but receives.

Yet the chapters are not naive about the risks of love in the transference. In *Transferential Love*, transference is analysed not as a false love but as a staged repetition of unconscious drama, capable of leading to either an impasse or a transformation. The analyst's task is not to love back in the usual sense, but to sustain the conditions under which the subject may encounter themselves through the Other.

Not all love is redemptive. Throughout this collection, love is portrayed as bordering on madness, destruction, and death. In *Dying of Love*, love is mourned, idealised, lost, and sometimes literally fatal. Literature, cinema, and music echo the ambivalence Freud and Klein already identified: that we love what we also hate, and hate what we cannot do without. Love kills and revives. In *Radiography of Seduction* and *Pornocracy*, the object of love becomes spectral, commodified, and made available on demand. Desire, when decoupled from the symbolic and reduced to repetition, loses its vitality. The chapters do not moralise this condition, but ask how we might reinject the erotic with ethical tension, with lack, with mystery. Not all love is good, but even perverse love teaches us about the fault lines of our subjectivity.

Love unfolds in time – too soon, too late, never enough. Several chapters, notably '*From Prehistoric to Futuristic Love*' and '*Internet Love,*' explore how our technological and evolutionary pasts and futures shape our capacity to desire. Love is not static; it adapts, fails, morphs. But the question remains: is there a core that persists beneath these changes?

Perhaps the core is this: that love calls us out of ourselves. As Fromm, Winnicott, and Badiou each suggest in different ways, to love is to risk. It is to let go of mastery, of fusion, of the illusion of self-completeness. *Love's Infinitives* – to long, to care, to wait, to mourn, to give – are all acts that require a decentring of the ego. That is why love hurts. That is also why it matters.

In composing this kaleidoscope of love, the intention was never to offer closure. Like desire itself, the chapters turn in circles, repeat motifs, and break off where something more might be said. But perhaps that is the only fitting form for love: a form that fragments and refracts, rather than subsumes. Love, in psychoanalytic terms, is always incomplete. It speaks through lapsus, dreams, symptoms, and songs. It shows itself not in definitions but in traces, in acts, in silences. These chapters have tried to remain faithful to that incompleteness, not to explain love, but to listen to what it does. Let this epilogue, then, not be an end, but an invitation: to think love again, to desire otherwise, to read between the lines of the heart.

Index

For Product Safety Concerns and Information please contact our EU representative GPSR@taylorandfrancis.com
Taylor & Francis Verlag GmbH, Kaufingerstraße 24, 80331 München, Germany

www.ingramcontent.com/pod-product-compliance
Ingram Content Group UK Ltd.
Pitfield, Milton Keynes, MK11 3LW, UK
UKHW022020180926
475701UK00005B/947

* 9 7 8 1 0 4 1 2 1 7 3 2 9 *